Praise for *Sacred Oils*

'A healer of extraordinary power, Felicity Warner
shares her considerable knowledge with warmth
and love. A book not to be missed.'

JUDY HALL, AUTHOR OF THE CRYSTAL BIBLE AND THE CRYSTAL COMPANION

'Working with the sacred oils demands sensitivity, experience,
insight, inspiration and deepest respect. These are all qualities
that I use to describe soul midwife, healer and author Felicity
Warner. Through this book, she empowers you to step safely and
powerfully into another healing dimension with the sacred oils.'

RHIANNON LEWIS, EDITOR OF THE INTERNATIONAL JOURNAL
OF CLINICAL AROMATHERAPY AND FOUNDER OF BOTANICA
INTERNATIONAL AROMATHERAPY CONFERENCES

T0035755

Praise for *The Soul Midwives' Handbook,* also by Felicity Warner

'A gift for bringing comfort and peace to
those who are about to pass away.'
DAILY EXPRESS

'The woman who wants to make dying more dignified.'
WOMAN'S WEEKLY

'In this moving book, Felicity has encapsulated the wisdom
of the ages into practical examples of how to BE with the
dying; how to honour and hold that sacred space for everyone
as they prepare to make the journey that we all must take.'
ANITA MOORJANI, AUTHOR OF *DYING TO BE ME*

'It is wonderful that Felicity Warner's Soul Midwives
now have a handbook for practical use. As vigiling
reclaims its rightful place at the bedside, The Soul
Midwives' Handbook *emerges as a useful and timely
tool for those who are called to this sacred work.'*
MEGORY ANDERSON PHD, AUTHOR OF *SACRED DYING*

'By providing loving and gentle support, Felicity and
the Soul Midwives support people to have the death
that they want. What could be more important?'
JON UNDERWOOD, PIONEER OF THE DEATH CAFE MOVEMENT

Sacred Oils

Also by Felicity Warner
and published by Hay House

Books

The Soul Midwives' Handbook (2011)

A Safe Journey Home (2011)

A Gentle Dying (2008)

Audio Digital Downloads and CDs

A Journey with Sacred Oils (2019)

Sacred Oils

Working with 20 Precious Oils to Heal Spirit and Soul

FELICITY WARNER

HAY HOUSE

Carlsbad, California • New York City
London • Sydney • New Delhi

Published in the United Kingdom by:
Hay House UK Ltd, The Sixth Floor, Watson House,
54 Baker Street, London W1U 7BU
Tel: +44 (0)20 3927 7290; Fax: +44 (0)20 3927 7291
www.hayhouse.co.uk

Published in the United States of America by:
Hay House Inc., PO Box 5100, Carlsbad, CA 92018-5100
Tel: (1) 760 431 7695 or (800) 654 5126
Fax: (1) 760 431 6948 or (800) 650 5115
www.hayhouse.com

Published in Australia by:
Hay House Australia Ltd, 18/36 Ralph St, Alexandria NSW 2015
Tel: (61) 2 9669 4299; Fax: (61) 2 9669 4144
www.hayhouse.com.au

Published in India by:
Hay House Publishers India, Muskaan Complex,
Plot No.3, B-2, Vasant Kunj, New Delhi 110 070
Tel: (91) 11 4176 1620; Fax: (91) 11 4176 1630
www.hayhouse.co.in

A catalogue record for this book is available from the British Library.

Tradepaper ISBN: 978-1-4019-7346-9
E-book ISBN: 978-1-78817-174-8

Printed in the United States of America

10 9 8 7 6 5 4 3 2 1

This book is dedicated to those who have kept
this sacred and ancient tradition alive.

*For those who have ears to hear and eyes to see
where the nous lies, there is the treasure.*

Go and catch a falling star,
Get with child a mandrake root,
Tell me where all past years are,
Or who cleft the devil's foot;
Teach me to hear mermaids singing,
Or to keep off envy's stinging,
And find
What wind
Serves to advance an honest mind.

If thou be'st born to strange sights,
Things invisible to see,
Ride ten thousand days and nights
Till age snow white hairs on thee;
Thou, when thou return'st, wilt tell me
All strange wonders that befell thee,
And swear
No where
Lives a woman true and fair.

If thou find'st one, let me know,
Such a pilgrimage were sweet;
Yet do not, I would not go,
Though at next door we might meet.
Though she were true when you met her,
And last till you write your letter,
Yet she
Will be
False, ere I come, to two, or three.

SONG: GO AND CATCH A FALLING STAR, JOHN DONNE

Contents

Acknowledgements

Without the loving and loyal support of my husband, Richard, this book might have remained a scattered collection of notes and diaries. In always choosing to take the path less travelled, my curiosity and passion for exploring the inner realms have made me a nomadic time-traveller of sorts rather than staying 'at home' to get the supper on the table and the ironing done. Richard ensures that our hearth is tended and warm, and that the cats, Zennor, Sorcha and Padstow, are fed.

I'd also like to thank all those who have helped me in other ways.

Michelle Pilley and her amazing team at Hay House; the intuitive and gentle Jane Struthers for weaving such magic; and my agent, Chelsey Fox, for supporting my work and for her constant encouragement.

My lovely daughters, Daisy and Lusea; my granddaughters, Matilda, Amelie and Beatrice, and the new baby on the way, for making me smile so much.

My dear PA, Samantha Martin, for being my loyal and fantastic gatekeeper.

My wonderful, compassionate and loving soul midwives, too many to mention personally, but especially Mandy, Dee, Krista, Wendy, Jude, Suzi, Michael and William, who give me endless love and support.

To my dear friends, including Mel Bailey and Buster for teaching me to ride; and to Sarah Peters, my oldest friend, who made flower perfumes with me when we were children.

To Sir John Tavener for opening portals through sound and energy; and to Lucy M. Boston for inspiring me with her writing and whole way of being.

To Lys De Grasse; and, of course, Mary Magdalene, the greatest teacher of all time.

Introduction

Essential oils have become familiar to many of us in recent decades. They can easily be bought online and in health-food shops, and can be used for everything from putting a few drops in a diffuser to scent a room to adding a combination of oils to a bath and dabbing some on a pillow to encourage restful sleep. Aromatherapists, who work professionally with the oils, use them to treat many ailments, both mental and physical.

Sacred oils are different. They're a small group of essential oils that, as their name suggests, have special energies and sacred properties. Some of them, such as Rose and Patchouli, may already be known to you (although possibly for different purposes), while you may be meeting others, such as Opoponax and Ravensara, for the first time. As you'll discover in *Sacred Oils*, I've worked with these oils for many years, especially in the course of my work as a soul midwife (a spiritual and holistic therapist for the dying). Almost all of these oils have an age-old lineage, which I describe in the book; although one of them is a very recent and valuable addition, whose time has come because its energy is now needed by the world.

Sacred Oils is divided into two parts. Part I describes how I was first introduced to sacred oils and how I became a part of the myrrhophore tradition – an ancient and secret group of women who work with the oils for the highest good of everyone. This section of the book also tells you how to work with the oils in meditation and how to call on them whenever you need their help.

In Part II, I describe the 20 oils that I've included in this book. I've not only given you practical information about them, but also their esoteric qualities and uses. There's also a guided meditation for each oil so that you can get to know it better. Finally, so you can see how they work, I've included a case study for each oil. Please note that some of the details in each case study have been changed to respect individuals' privacy.

At the end of the book are some resources that I hope you'll find helpful, including a short bibliography and a list of oil suppliers.

If you're new to sacred oils, I hope this book will serve as an inspiring introduction to these very valuable and spiritual entities. If you've already met some or all of these sacred oils, I hope this book will deepen and enrich your experience of them.

PART I

Working with the Oils

CHAPTER 1

My Own Story of Working with the Oils

'There is a Spirit that is mind and life, light and truth and vast spaces. It contains all works and desires and all perfumes and all tastes. It enfolds the whole universe, and in silence is loving to all.'

CHANDOGYA UPANISHAD, *THE VEDIC SCRIPTURES*

From my earliest years, I've been drawn to essential oils. As a child, I loved smelling my grandmother's hankies that had been rinsed in lavender oil. I spent many hours in the garden picking scented flowers and packing them into bottles to make perfumes for the fairies.

Even then, the smells were an intoxicating mystery to me. How did a violet get its perfume? What gave rose petals their gentle scent? And why could I smell the velvet-soft vanilla notes of warm wallflowers in the Sun? These aromas touched me deeply and often inspired curious thoughts, opening a doorway into a secret world.

Aged about four, while my mother baked rock cakes, I spent hours picking and arranging brightly coloured nasturtiums. I lost track of time, absorbed by their peppery scent and dazzling colours, which seemed as bright as the Sun. They lifted my spirits and took me to another place.

I was soon making simple creams and floral waters. I wanted to learn everything I could about scent, but no one seemed to know much, other than explaining the science of oils and molecules, and how our sense of smell works (which seemed pathetic in comparison to dogs), so I decided to ask the flowers themselves. I asked them who and what they were. I was surprised to get some very 'enlightening' answers from them.

How do you begin a conversation with a plant? I began by closing my eyes tight, smelling a particular plant and then intuitively sensing a response. Every plant seemed to have a different voice and teaching to share. My mother once found me lying in her prized herbaceous border talking to a clump of larkspur. Even now, I remember how interesting their conversations were. No wonder my mother always described me as being rather 'fey'.

A Meeting in Copenhagen

My first introduction to the world of sacred oils came when I was 15 and living in Copenhagen, Denmark. I was given the space and freedom to explore all sorts of interesting and diverse activities; as long as I was safe, my mother didn't mind what I was doing.

I made friends with an opera singer called Ida who lived in the next-door flat, which was crammed with books, ceramics, paintings, dried herbs and plants. Her stimulating company encouraged me on my spiritual pathway.

We talked of angels, the poet William Blake, metaphysical poets, magic and alchemy – and she loaned me the most exciting books I'd ever read. Ida had many interesting acquaintances, mainly musicians, writers and artists, and one day she took me to visit a friend who lived in an austere block of flats on the edge of the city.

Lys was a funky old lady dressed in black with long grey hair and bright red specs. She was tough and feisty. Her flat was exquisite – her furniture was painted in soft, chalky blues and greys, her floors were a soft wash of silvery paint, and all the walls were lined with rows of tiny bottles and hundreds of books. It had the atmosphere of a sanctuary or hermitage and it felt like home to me.

We had camomile tea and then she brought out some bottles for us to smell. I felt nervous. She opened each bottle with reverence, carefully unscrewing the cap, lifting the bottle to her nose, breathing in deeply, seeming in a reverie, her eyes closed. She didn't speak but had a look of rapt pleasure on her face. I sat in awe, reminded of Japanese tea rituals.

Eventually, Lys handed me a tiny bright blue glass bottle. Cautiously, I took a light sniff, then a deeper, longer one that filled my nostrils. Wow! What was this smell? My nose twitched and tingled. Was it liquid fire? Ice? Arctic air? Then I saw colours. Deep aqua, silver streaks, magenta flashes. Not only did I smell something I'd never smelled before, but I was also seeing colours in my head.

As I inhaled deeper, I could feel myself crunching in deep crystalline snow up to my knees, listening to trees moaning in the wind. I was walking with a small child towards a house with a red door...

Lys called me back gently, asking if I'd enjoyed the smell.

Back in the reality of her sitting room, I didn't have the language (or the confidence) to explain my experience, but she could see that something had happened to me.

Rather like Alice in Wonderland, everything was getting curiouser and curiouser. I felt wobbly and slightly dizzy, and so another bottle was whipped off a shelf and waved under my nose. This one brought me straight back into the present and my legs felt as heavy as lead.

This was the first of many visits and I got to know Lys well over the next three years. When I was experiencing a new oil with her, she would always listen attentively, without interrupting, watching me for any micro-expressions and reading my light body – the sum of a person's energetic layers, from the densest physical body to the subtlest spiritual body; although I didn't know about things like that then. This was the beginning of my training. Gently, and very cautiously, Lys revealed more.

Although she was a retired psychotherapist, the oils were her real life's work. She blended them or sourced others from far-flung and obscure places around the world. Lys was the most reclusive person I've ever met, yet charming and kind. She was extremely articulate and a very good listener, but secretive and guarded when it came to the oils.

Myrrhophores

Gradually, Lys revealed herself to be a myrrhophore or 'mistress of the oils' – a description that she'd been given by her own teacher. She explained that her lineage could be traced back to the myrrhophores (women bearing myrrh), who belonged to pre-biblical Egyptian temple traditions.

These temple priestesses were trained from puberty in the healing arts. They were picked for their sensitivity to energy, for their sharp 'noses', and for their ability to recognize the most potent and powerful aromatic oils. They were master energy healers, trained to work with the extreme energy of these oils. Their formidable skills healed not the body, but the soul.

Lys taught me that this is an esoteric (hidden) tradition, oblique and camouflaged to deflect from the power it carries. 'It's dangerous to have knowledge without wisdom' was one of her mantras.

She observed that I had a nose like a sniffer dog and a snake-like ability to sense vibration. These were two essential talents for becoming a myrrhophore, but still not enough for her to decide to begin teaching me. I had to prove that I was physically robust enough to be a vessel for the high energies that I'd be working with. This couldn't be taught, only discovered through a series of initiations and much challenging practical work.

And so I began my apprenticeship. I was tested to the limits to see how much energy I could 'hold' and if I could discharge it when I was full (holding high energy for too long can make you ill).

This was the beginning of a long and sometimes gruelling phase, during which I might struggle up a level or so and then be totally blocked for a time while I absorbed the knowledge I was being given. Like peeling an onion, there were layers upon layers of understanding about the way the oils worked, and most of them were veiled in hermetic and alchemical-like symbolism.

For three years, until I left Denmark to return to England, Lys and I worked with the oils. When I left, she gave me a silver chest for my oils and a hand-made leather notebook as my oils grimoire, in which she'd written, in large, flowing handwriting, 'Song' by John Donne. (You'll find it at the front of this book.)

She then anointed me on my forehead with an oil, whose composition had been channelled from the discarnate priestesses of lineage, to begin my work. I still don't know what was in it, but the aroma – something between recently disturbed earth from the forest floor and the smell of ancient churches – will linger in my memory forever.

Initiation into the Myrrhophore Lineage

You need another myrrhophore in the physical realm to initiate you into the lineage before embarking on out-of-body training in the etheric temples. You gain entry to the temples through dreams, trances, sound, symbols, vibrations and, of course, smell, taught by the oils themselves because they're teachers of divine intelligence. The training is arduous and all of my teachers are now in spirit. Even now, my energy field is constantly tested and challenged at every level to ensure that I can work with safety and integrity.

I've always been very sensitive to atmospheres and my surroundings. When I was a child, I only had to walk into a room of people I didn't know to be violently sick or come out in a rash. I could tune in to everything, both good and bad. Even then, I could sense another person's energy and read it, which was exhausting.

It eventually affected my health. I had eczema, asthma, a grumbling appendix throughout my early years and I'd be struck down by sudden fevers. During both my pregnancies I developed severe pre-eclampsia – a dangerous condition partly caused by pregnancy-induced high blood pressure. I also have many allergies.

I have a fragile but intense energy field and my work with oils has intensified this. Before working with others, I've had to learn to cure myself, rebalancing my chakras and aura on a daily basis.

Why I've Written This Book

Information on working with the sacred oils is hard to find and very little is written down. This is because the teaching is part of an oral tradition passed from mistress (or master) to student. So, why am I writing a book without betraying this secret tradition?

The oils themselves have decreed that the time is right, because they're here to be of greater benefit to humanity. Many of their teachings are ready to be shared in order to help expand global consciousness. They know that their gentle but potent healing is needed in these challenging times.

For the past few years, I've been working with the oils in my soul midwifery work, teaching other soul midwives and healers about how these extraordinary oils can transform *all* journeys in life, not just at the end of life. New oils are being channelled to help planet Earth as she shifts and increases her own vibration. Pure vials of base oil are being filled with new and vibrant energies, and the reasons for this are quietly being revealed.

The depth of these teachings is still being taught to me as I commit myself deeper into service of the lineage. I take a daily vow to hold these teachings in my heart. In addition, I promise to learn, contemplate and protect this knowledge in order to share it with those who'll both honour the teachings and use them for the highest good.

I hope that everyone reading this book will feel inspired to work with the oils, opening their spirits and souls to the extraordinary wisdom that the oils possess.

CHAPTER 2

The Myrrhophore Tradition

"'Dear Lucius," he said, "how blessed you are that the
great Goddess has graciously deigned to honour you in
this way. There is no time to waste. The day for which
you prayed so earnestly has dawned. The many-named
Goddess orders me to initiate you into her holy mysteries."

He took me by the hand and led me courteously to the doors
of the vast temple. He went to the adytum and took out
two or three books written in characters unknown to me:
some of them animal hieroglyphics, some of them ordinary
letters, having their tops and tails wreathed in knots or
rounded like wheels or tangled together like vine tendrils.
From these books he read me instructions for providing
the necessary clothes and accessories for my initiation.
I at once went to my friends the priests and asked
them to buy part of what I needed, sparing no
expense: the rest I went to buy myself.'

APULEIUS, *The Golden Ass*

The myrrhophore tradition grew from 'celestial medicine' that was practised in the temples of ancient Egypt. Celestial medicine was based on the ritualistic relationship between planetary agreements (known as the law of similar) and the signatures of body constitution, ailments and the remedies that would heal them. It was a complex but powerful form of healing.

Myrrhophores, also known as myrrh bearers or mistresses of the oils, were priestesses skilled in helping people who were approaching death; they also gave healing when necessary. Their primary healing work was to realign people with their true soul essence and to heal the wounds in the soul caused by events not only in this life, but also in previous lives. As their name implies, they used oils to do this.

These women were the daughters of priestesses, so were part of a sacred lineage. Their temple training began when they reached puberty, at which point they were taught to work with energy through a series of initiations in alchemy, energy, and death and dying (transition) work. In order to ensure that the heart of the mysteries was both maintained and in safe hands, the faith, devotion and integrity of the myrrhophores were constantly being tested. The most famous myrrhophore was Mary Magdalene, and the Bible contains many instances of both her work and that of her sister myrrhophores, especially during crucifixion.

The Modern Attributes of Myrrhophores

Myrrhophores are still healer priestesses in one form or another and are well practised in energy medicine. They use their inner vision (the eyes of spirit) to read energy fields, as well as to assess the core energetic system of their clients, so as to heal and make whole the spirit and soul.

One of the first lessons that a myrrhophore has to learn is to access the *nous*, which is the wisdom of the heart and soul. It's the basis of everything we learn and understand in working with the soul. It's the divine intelligence that lives within us and is channelled from God. The Greeks called this *metis*: an intuitive intelligence that's often attributed to women. Sacred oils connect us to the energy of the Divine.

CHAPTER 3

The Origins and Traditions of Working with Sacred Oils

'In the midst of the Elysian Fields they were to find a golden city with emerald ramparts, ivory pavements and cinnamon gates. Around the walls flowed a river of perfumes one hundred cubits in width and deep enough to swim in. From this river rose an odorous mist, which enveloped the whole place and shed a refreshing and fragrant dew. There were to be, besides, in this fortunate city, three hundred and sixty-five fountains of honey and five hundred of the sweetest essences.'

EUGENE RIMMEL, *THE BOOK OF PERFUMES*

A romatic plants have been used in medicines and rituals for at least 70,000 years. Traces of plants, seeds and resins have been discovered by archaeologists excavating the ancient temples and tombs of many early civilizations, including the ancient Egyptians, Sumerians, Babylonians and Chaldeans. They all used plants for healing, and small particles of lavender, spikenard, myrrh and sandalwood have been discovered in their tombs.

An Ancient Legacy

Early medical systems, such as Ayurvedic, Tibetan and Chinese medicine, were mainly plant-based and the systems were applied by doctors/priests. Vedic literature that was written in about 2000BCE in India mentions many hundreds of aromatic substances, including sandalwood and myrrh. They were not only valued as fragrances, but also for their therapeutic and ceremonial uses. In China, at roughly the same time, the *Yellow Emperor's Book of Internal Medicine* listed plants, including ginger, that were used in both medicine and religion.

Ancient Egypt is one of the civilizations most closely associated with its extensive use of oils. Papyri from about 2800BCE mentioned medicinal herbs, and some from about 2000BCE described oils, perfumes and incense.

Mummification

One of the best-known uses of oils in ancient times was in mummification. The ancient Egyptians were extremely skilled in the art of preserving bodies after death, rubbing a variety of aromatic gums, including cedar and myrrh, on bodies before they were mummified. The resins from these gums were antibacterial and fungicidal, thereby preventing the bodies from decaying. Jars of essential oils have been found in the tombs of pharaohs.

The ancient Egyptians believed that there was a strong link between scent and healing, and their god Nefertem had rulership of both. Disagreeable smells were associated with impurity and pleasant aromas suggested that sacred entities were nearby.

Modern Times

Essential oils as we know them today are comparatively modern, dating back to the last 600 years or so. Rose oil is thought to be the first oil created as a byproduct of making rosewater, which was used for perfumery and flavouring food. The copper stills involved were very small and primitive, and so the amounts of oil produced were tiny.

Essential oils are highly concentrated volatile oils found in various parts of plants, including the petals, leaves, bark and roots. The oils are extracted using several different methods:

◊   steam distillation

◊   solvent extraction

◊   resin harvesting

◊ enfleurage, in which essential oils from petals are pressed into odourless fats that then absorb the oils

◊ maceration, the oldest method of all, in which fragrant petals are soaked in oil for a period of time before being strained and bottled.

The therapeutic use of essential oils is often referred to as 'aromatherapy', a term that was first used in 1928 by Gattefossé, who was a French chemist. During his work in his family's perfumery business he began to explore the healing qualities of essential oils, which can be used to treat both physical and emotional ailments.

How Modern Aromatherapy Differs from Sacred Oils

Just about the only thing that links modern aromatherapy with the practice of working with sacred oils is that they both use essential oils. Otherwise, they have almost nothing in common. Modern aromatherapy is largely a smell-sensory experience, in which the aromatherapist chooses oils for their relaxing qualities. The smell of the oils stimulates the olfactory nerves in the nose. In turn, these calm the limbic system in the brain, bringing a sense of pleasure, release and relaxation.

Clinical aromatherapy, which is more of a specialist practice used in hospitals and hospices, uses essential oils to treat infections (many oils have antibacterial qualities), promote the healing of wounds, increase the flow of lymph through the body following surgery or for simple massage. An aromatherapist will take a client's medical history before working with them. They'll also ensure that the treatment room is warm, a couch is available for massage and that clean towels are at the ready. They may use familiar oils such as Lavender, Bergamot or Rose Geranium for many purposes: massage, oil burners to scent the room, room sprays (with added water) and electric diffusers. They may also put a few drops on a client's temples or use them as pillow sprays to aid relaxing sleep.

The practice of sacred oils is very different. Its roots are based in ancient shamanic magic and ritual practice (enabling us to contact our guides or power animals). The smell of the oil being used isn't important or valuable in the treatments – it's the oil's spiritual and esoteric qualities that are important. Myrrhophores don't use sacred oils for massage.

Modern aromatherapy oils are rather like opening a simple, ready-mixed watercolour paintbox and painting a beautiful picture with them. Sacred oils, by comparison, are like painting a religious icon using ground pigments made from precious stones and minerals, blending them with egg yolk and gold leaf, to create a spiritual picture that will last for hundreds of years.

In summary, sacred oils are used in the following ways:

◊ Meditation

◊ Healing soul wounds

◊ Expanding and scanning the energy field

◊ Cleansing the aura

◊ Anointing

◊ Ritual

◊ Psychopomp work

◊ Opening the third eye

◊ Accessing past-life information

◊ Creating sacred space

◊ For vision and prophecy

Why Some Oils Are Sacred

Although nearly all oils have some therapeutic value, only those that resonate energetically with the spirit and soul are deemed sacred.

The Soul and the Spirit

The soul is our link to the Divine and the eternal part of ourselves that survives into eternity. It carries our consciousness with it after death. The spirit is the ego/personality aspect of ourselves that contains the essence of who we are in this lifetime. When we heal the soul we're healing problems that may have followed us from previous lifetimes and may possibly extend into the future. In contrast, healing the spirit involves healing us in the here and now on a spiritual level.

The Sense of Smell and the Seat of the Soul

The ancient Egyptians believed that the sense of smell and the ability to intuit the effects of smells are the most important sensory abilities that we have. Why? Because they knew that the inhalation and energy absorption of oils can increase our energetic frequency by stimulating the pineal gland.

This gland, which is a tiny mass of nerve tissue buried deep within the back of the brain, is thought to be the seat of the soul and the divine connector to enlightenment within the body. It attracts energy from the highest source and is governed by the crown chakra (*see page 42*). Energy carries light and information, and the *nous* (the wisdom of the heart and soul) is activated and expanded by this invisible energy.

Throughout history, certain oils have been used to invoke altered states of consciousness and initiate individuals into various spiritual traditions. To anoint (from the Latin *inunctum*, meaning to smear with oil) someone is to make them sacred, to set them apart, offer a ritualized blessing and dedicate them to serve a higher spiritual purpose.

Coronation Oil

Essential oils have other uses, too. Whenever a British monarch is crowned, at the climax of the ceremony they're anointed with a special blend of oils, to draw down divine sovereignty to the new king or queen. This is such a sacred act that it's conducted beneath a canopy, out of sight of the thousands of people who attend the coronation. The special oil is prepared in advance and then consecrated, before being placed in the ampulla, which is a gold vessel in the shape of an eagle. At the appropriate moment during the coronation service, the oil is poured out through the beak of the eagle-shaped ampulla into the anointing spoon, which is used to anoint the sovereign's hands, breast and head.

The exact recipe for the oil is kept secret, but it's based on one from the 17th century. It consists of sesame seed and olive oils, with oils of rose, jasmine, orange, cinnamon, musk, civet and ambergris. Although the latter three are now extremely hard to source, the blend of the other oils creates a very powerful, highly energized oil that has a smell that isn't quite of this world. Rose, orange and jasmine oils all have links to the angelic realms, carrying an extremely high frequency.

Other Essential Oils

The vast majority of essential oils are generally used in a non-sacred way, such as eucalyptus for helping us to breathe when we have a cold. Some essential oils, such as Fragonia™, lavender and Rose, are common in modern aromatherapy, yet also have sacred powers. Patchouli, for example, can be used at a simple level as a perfume; in clinical aromatherapy for fighting serious infections because of its antibacterial qualities; and for exploring past-life memory in its sacred use. It only becomes a sacred oil when a sacred space is created and an intention is set to work with it for sacred purposes.

The Oils in This Book

The 20 oils that I've chosen for this book represent just a few in the sacred repertoire. The oils themselves dictated their inclusion by being robust and colourful, and by giving the sense that they wanted to be written about. Others that I'd planned to include became ephemeral and hard to focus on. As such, they drifted slightly out of view and were difficult to contact during meditation. I was therefore guided to take the hint that they wanted to remain hidden and aloof and aren't yet ready to share their gifts.

The oils that I've described in this book are:

◊ **Angelica:** A master teacher

◊ **Cedarwood Atlas:** Strength of spirit

◊ **Elemi:** Letting go, surrender

◊ **Fragonia™:** For transitions of every kind

◊ **Frankincense:** Aligning spirit and soul with the Divine

◊ **Galbanum:** Opening portals, psychopomp

◊ **Holy Basil:** Reconnecting with the divine life force

◊ **Marigold:** Vision and prophecy

◊ **Myrrh:** Wisdom and forgiveness

◊ **Myrtle:** Gatekeeper of the Sacred Threshold for summoning the Muse

◊ **Opoponax:** Shape-shifting and shape-borrowing

◊ **Palo Santo:** Protection

◊ **Patchouli:** Grounding

◊ **Ravensara:** Healing soul wounds

◊ **Rose:** Love and learning to love yourself and your inner child

◊ **Sandalwood:** Meditation and listening deeply

◊ **Silver Fir:** Journeying and accessing personal power

◊ **Spikenard:** The Consolamentum oil – a glimpse of Paradise

◊ **Violet Leaf:** Extreme grief

◊ **Yarrow:** Sensitivity, fear and soul wounds

These oils are sacred for many reasons:

◊ They're powerful and divine intelligences

◊ They're energy and light manifested in matter

◊ They're sacred tools of consciousness

◊ They have energy signatures that resonate with the human soul and spirit

◊ They can help us to project consciousness for use in healing others and to become multidimensional

◊ They can prompt visionary experiences and take us back to past lives

◊ They're oracular and can show us the future

◊ They can be used as tools for mass consciousness

◊ They heal the light body and the soul

I believe that sacred oils are energies that have originated from other dimensions, including other star systems and galaxies. They have come in service to help humankind to evolve its consciousness. In Part II, I describe the karmic roots of each oil, to give a fuller understanding of its origins and power.

CHAPTER 4

How to Begin Working with the Oils

*'Following in the footsteps of the wise elders who
have practised this sacred art before me, I ask
to be shown where my work may be done.*

*I offer unconditional support, love,
connection, depth and companionship
to those who ask me to help them as
they work with the sacred oils.'*

INVOCATION TO THE OILS, TRADITIONAL

Although it may be tempting to begin your work with sacred oils immediately, there are several steps you need to take first, so that you know what you're doing and you can establish a strong relationship with the oils.

You will need:

◊ A journal or notebook in which you can record your experiences with the oils – only use it for your work with sacred oils, and try to include the date and time of each entry in case you need to refer to these at a later date

◊ A pen or pencil

◊ A clean bottle

◊ A sticky label

◊ Carrier oil

◊ Your chosen sacred oil

Keeping a Journal

A journal is a wonderful tool for recording any impressions, ideas and inspirations that come when you work or meditate with an oil. Any notebook will do, but a beautiful one that's dedicated to your sacred work is even nicer. Remember that anything you write (or draw) should be for your eyes only. Important messages from the oils (which may come to you in intuitive ideas and symbols) are often only revealed when we look back on what we've jotted down during several sessions of working with an oil.

Bottles and Carrier Oils

In order to work with sacred oils, you'll need some clean glass bottles into which you can put your blends of carrier and essential oils. These are usually small 5ml or 10ml bottles made of dark brown or blue glass. They're available from a variety of suppliers (*see Stockists*). You should always use a clean bottle when mixing up a new blend, so it's not contaminated by traces of the previous mixture.

Sacred oils should always be blended with a carrier oil. You can buy all sorts of carrier oils, but the one I always use is organic rapeseed oil. It's so thick that it's like putting the sacred oils on a velvet cushion.

Preparing Your Oil

1. Pour 10ml of your carrier oil into a clean bottle.

2. Add a few drops (I suggest five drops) of your chosen oil.

3. Replace the lid and shake the bottle to blend the mixture.

4. Write the name of the sacred oil onto a label and place it onto the front of the bottle.

Calling in a Gatekeeper

Before you begin working with the oils, you need to work with a gatekeeper oil to protect you as you work. We all need a gatekeeper to guide and protect us whenever we're using our consciousness outside the physical realm. I suggest that you use Myrtle (see page 145) as your gatekeeper oil, because its energy is strong and compassionate. She'll filter the energies that are attracted to you and be the guardian of your space. Sit quietly with Myrtle, smell the oil and use the meditation she gives (see page 150) to ask her to become the gatekeeper for you.

We also have our own gatekeepers (special guides) who act as our guardians, and who filter the many energies and entities that roam the ether, challenging them if they try to enter our spiritual space. We need to work with a gatekeeper oil because it will understand the energies that are attracted by the vibrations of oils, which are usually fine and high. A gatekeeper oil can also help us to transmute very high energies into a level that we can easily work with without becoming overloaded – something that can happen when we work with an energy that's too high for us.

Greeting an Oil for the First Time

When you work with an oil for the first time, you need to become familiar with its particular field of energy by meditating with it and asking it some questions. Before you begin, prepare your oil (see page 31) and have your journal and a pen or pencil by your side.

1. Sit in a quiet place indoors or outdoors where you'll be totally undisturbed.

2. Close your eyes and consciously breathe slowly and deeply until you feel centred.

3. Ground yourself by imagining deep, strong roots, like those of a tree, growing from your body deep into the earth. These will help to anchor you and stop you from 'flying away'.

4. Visualize a sphere of bright, protective white light completely surrounding you, reaching below your feet, above your head and around your back. Feel yourself enclosed within it.

5. State your intention – what you want to achieve during this session, such as understanding the oil's energy.

6. Take your vial of oil, remove the cap and smell the oil.

7. Ask the oil for its permission to work with it and receive its wisdom.

8. Allow the oil to speak to you. Explore the feelings and emotions that you experience, paying attention to any shapes or symbols that appear in your mind. Talk to the oil.

9. You're now ready to ask it the following questions:

    ◊ What can you teach me?

    ◊ What do I need to release?

    ◊ What gift do you have for me?

10. Take note of anything that transpires, including all that you feel and see.

11. Check your physical body to see if you have any sensations, such as warmth or tingling.

12. When you've gathered as much information as you can (or if you're ready to end the meditation), give thanks to the oil and focus once again on your breath, then gently come back to the present.

13. Ground yourself once again and make notes in your journal about anything that you experienced.

Listen with your heart (rather than your head) to understand what the oil's telling you. Write down the information as soon as you can. If you're given a symbol to work with, jot this down, too. If your intention isn't stated, there'll only be limited power for your work. Sometimes oils that are connecting with us through our *nous* will let us know if they'd like to work with us to teach us deeper mysteries.

Connecting with an Oil

Pick a time when you won't be disturbed and choose an oil that you'd like to become more familiar with. Before you begin, prepare your oil (*see page 31*) and have your journal and a pen or pencil by your side.

1. Make yourself comfortable and do some deep breathing to put yourself into a quiet and reflective mood.

2. Now, open the bottle and smell the oil.

3. Notice the sensations you immediately experience. Jot them down in your journal.

4. When you're connected with the spirit of the oil, ask its permission to work with it. Within sacred work, it's required etiquette to ask permission from the source of wisdom you're working with.

5. Set your intention.

Preparing for a Guided Meditation

In Part II, you'll find a guided meditation for each of the 20 sacred oils included in this book. Each meditation will help you to tune in to the energy of that oil, so that you can begin to attune yourself to its frequency and absorb its wisdom. You'll find it easier to work with a guided meditation if you record it first, so that you can listen to it in a relaxed state, without having to refer constantly back to the book.

Work in the same way as described earlier for connecting with an oil. You may want to repeat the guided meditation more than once, so you can really get to know the personality and qualities of a specific oil.

Calling in a Teacher Oil

'I am Isis, mistress of the whole land. I am she who rises in the Dog Star. I am she who separated the heaven from the Earth. I have instructed mankind in the mysteries. I have pointed out their paths to the stars. I have ordered the course of the sun and the Moon. I am queen of the rivers and winds and sea. I have brought together men and women. I gave mankind their laws and ordained what no one can alter. I have made justice more powerful than silver and gold. I have caused truth to be considered beautiful.

I am she who is called the goddess of women. I, Isis, am all that has been, that is or shall be, no mortal man hath ever me unveiled. The fruit which I have brought forth is the sun.'

INSCRIPTION FROM ISIS'S TEMPLE AT SAIS

Some oils have taken on the role of 'teacher' as part of their own service to the Divine. They willingly invite you to work and learn with them, teaching you through meditation.

Invoking a Teacher Oil

1. Make a sacred space in the room where you'll meditate. You might wish to decorate it with fresh flowers or play beautiful music to make a temple in your home dedicated to the work.

2. Ask to be connected with the highest essence of the oil you want to work with as you begin your meditation.

3. Either hold the bottle containing the oil and sniff from the bottle or pour a couple of drops onto the palm of your hand and sniff the aroma from there.

4. Once you feel a connection has been made, you can ask questions of the oil:

   ◊ Ask for the oil's sigil (write it down in your journal immediately after you've finished the meditation).

   ◊ Ask for the oil's sacred sound.

   ◊ Ask how you can serve the oil.

   ◊ Ask what you need to release and understand.

5. Remember to hear with your heart. Try not to over-analyse or over-rationalize the information you're given.

6. Make a vow to meditate and connect with this teacher oil for 28 days (one lunar month), fully committing to the process.

7. Write in your journal exactly what you experience and feel each time. It's likely that only after the 28 days have elapsed will these journal posts make any sense.

Entering the Etheric Temples

After working for some time with a master teacher oil, you'll be invited to enter the etheric temples for further initiation.

In his book *Egyptian Myths and Mysteries*, Rudolf Steiner suggested that any temple built in Greece in honour of a god, such as Poseidon or Aphrodite, was actually the physical embodiment of that god. So if someone could tune in to the frequency of the temple, they'd be able to connect with the god, too.

When I first began my etheric temple training, I'd visit healing temples in my dreams. I was told that I wouldn't always be conscious of what I was taught in the temple, but codes of light, already within me, would be ignited. I'd be able to download information that would be stored and released when needed. Oils are the physical manifestation of the intelligences they're created from and their temples all reflect this, resonating with these energies.

My gatekeeper taught me always to be vigilant and alert, and to make contact with the oils quietly, with humility and impeccable manners at all times.

CHAPTER 5

Key Techniques and Practices

'Not all the water in the rough rude sea
Can wash the balm off from an anointed king.'
WILLIAM SHAKESPEARE, *RICHARD II*, ACT 3, SCENE 2

Remember that each oil has the power (and choice) to initiate you into the deeper mysteries. If you aren't ready, or of the right heart, it will only work with you at a basic level until you prove your commitment. It's when we experience these moments of enlightenment that our lives are irreversibly changed and our reality shifts. This is initiation.

A Simple Guide to the Chakras

The human body has seven major chakras, which run in a line from the crown of the head to the base of the spine. Each chakra is an energy centre that affects the surrounding area of the body. Although we can't see them at a physical level, many people can sense them with their hands. They feel like spinning wheels of energy when they're functioning healthily.

Here's a simple guide to the position of each chakra in the body, the areas of the body each one governs, the colour or colours associated with it and the sacred oils that have a particular affinity with it.

Base Chakra

Position on the body: Perineum (area between anus and genitals)

Sites of energy: Feet, ankles, legs, knees, thighs, large intestine

Oils: Cedarwood Atlas, Myrrh, Opoponax, Palo Santo, Patchouli, Yarrow

Colour: Red

Sacral Chakra

Position on the body: Sexual organs and upwards towards the navel

Sites of energy: All fluid functions of the body; ovaries, testes, uterus

Oils: Rose, Sandalwood

Colour: Orange

Solar Plexus Chakra

Position on the body: Between the navel and centre of the solar plexus

Sites of energy: Pancreas, adrenals

Oils: Fragonia, Rose

Colour: Yellow

Heart Chakra

Position on the body: The heart area

Sites of energy: Heart, thymus, immune system

Oils: Angelica, Myrrh, Rose, Spikenard

Colour: Emerald green and rose pink

Throat Chakra

Position on the body: The throat region at the base of the neck

Sites of energy: Thyroid gland, lungs, vocal cords, jaw, breath

Oils: Myrrh

Colour: Blue

Brow (or Third Eye) Chakra

Position on the body: Between and just below the eyes

Sites of energy: Pituitary gland, left eye, base of the skull

Oils: Frankincense, Marigold, Myrtle, Silver Fir

Colour: Indigo

Crown Chakra

Position on the body: Crown of the head

Sites of energy: Right eye, cerebral cortex, pineal gland, upper skull, skin

Oils: Elemi, Frankincense, Galbanum, Holy Basil, Ravensara, Sandalwood, Violet Leaf

Colour: Violet, white and gold

Creating Sacred Space

To set the scene for working with sacred oils you need to prepare a sacred space. This creates the physical and psychic boundaries for your work. It also helps you to draw your focus inwards and to renew your spiritual connection, so you can receive higher guidance.

You can create a sacred space anywhere in your home – a spare bedroom, a corner of your sitting room, or by creating a simple altar on a windowsill or in an alcove. It can also be done outside. Decorate this space with objects that delight your senses, such as cushions, candles, sacred pictures of spiritual guides and teachers, beautiful shells and crystals, and some shallow dishes for your oils. A comfortable chair that supports your back while you meditate is a good idea.

Try to spend time every day in your sacred space. Set the intention that it's your sanctuary – a place for you to learn and connect. Light a candle, tone – by saying something like om or a mantra – and use a simple mantra or prayer to open and close your space each day.

If you're working away from home, you can create a temporary sacred space simply through the power of intention. Declare that a sacred space opens when you're ready to begin and then closes again after the sacred work has been completed. You can do this by saying, 'I ask for divine blessing to open a sacred space for this work and ask that it be held open for the highest good and that it be closed down again, with love, when the work is complete.'

Asking for a Symbol or Sigil

Some knowledge is too complex to be committed to language and the written word. Instead, it can be understood much better when it's represented by symbols or sigils. The word 'sigil' comes from the Latin *sigillum*, which means 'seal', as in the wax seals that were once applied to letters and documents. 'Sigil' can also mean a spiritual device or talisman.

When we want to begin a deep conversation with an oil, we need to ask it for a symbol that we can know it by – a sort

43

of password. The oil will channel a sigil to you that connects with your own energy field, which is why two people will have different sigils for the same oil. The sigil that an oil channels to you is unique to you.

Vibration

Each oil has its own vibrational signature. *The Kybalion*, a book on hermetic philosophy that was originally published in 1908 and claimed to be the essence of the teachings of Hermes Trismegistus, says that nothing rests – everything moves and everything vibrates. Through vibration, we learn the sacred principal ability to convert energy into mass and back into energy with the mind. In order to discover this, the myrrhophore has to learn to balance the aura perfectly. In the ancient temples, this technique was taught to all initiates, sometimes taking a lifetime to accomplish.

We now pollute our bodies with junk food and alcohol, we don't exercise enough, we're exposed to electrical and chemical toxins, and nor do we breathe properly. However, the frequencies of the oils will all help us to overcome these obstacles, so we can balance our auras again.

Sound Signatures

Each oil has its own sound signature, which it will transmit to you during meditation. Tone this sound to bring you into resonance with this oil. The tones might sound strange, often like long syllables rather than musical notes.

The easiest way to begin toning is to sing vowel sounds ('aaah', 'eeee', 'iiii', 'oooo' and 'uuuu') as loudly, and in whichever key, as feels right. The idea is to produce raw sound, not music. It's best done in private, so that you don't feel inhibited by the knowledge that others are listening to you. The sounds have the effect of opening up your chakras, which expands your energy field, enabling you to match your vibration with the frequency of the oil. As you tone, your voice may begin to rise or fall, opening out into grunting or yawning sounds.

Celebrate these toning sounds, because this technique is an essential part of linking into the energy of an oil.

Opening the Third Eye

Oils affect our personal frequency, so it's normal to experience unusual phenomena as a result of using them. This is because the oils help to open the third eye, which is the brow chakra.

It's a common experience to smell roses while making contact with angels, whether through prayer or meditation. Roses vibrate at the highest frequency of any flower, so angels, who also have a very high vibrational energy, find it easier to connect with these flowers than with any other. It's been found that Rose essential oil vibrates at 320 megahertz (320 million cycles per second), whereas the frequency of a healthy human brain is between 72 and 90 megahertz, and a healthy body frequency is between 62 and 72 megahertz.

When invoking an oil that they have chosen to work with, many people call their ancestors, spirit helpers and guides with a sacred song. You can ask all of these spirit guides for their help, love and guidance in gratitude for the sacred work that will begin. Ask that what occurs will be for the highest good of all life, everywhere.

Most of us can naturally sense energies through our hands, but we also have the potential to 'see' a person's energy field and core soul energies. Most healers can be trained to do this, but it usually requires you to have your own radar fine-tuned in order to see beyond the normal field. You fine-tune and expand your inner radar by keeping your energy field (your aura) pristine. This can be done in several different ways: by balancing your chakras on a daily basis; imagining light filling up your body; or imagining yourself taking a shower under a golden rain of light.

Using Sacred Oils to Help Others

Sacred oils can be used to help others in a number of ways:

Opening the Hand Chakras

It's the minor chakras in our hands that enable us to scan someone's energy field. If you're new to scanning, or want to ensure that your hand chakras are open before you begin, here's a simple exercise that I teach on my courses. You may prefer to practise it in private before you start scanning auras, so you can get used to how it feels to activate the minor chakras in your hands. Also, you'll find that the more you practise this exercise, the more quickly your hand chakras will open. Eventually, you'll be able to feel them opening at the appropriate time without having to do this exercise at all.

1. Stand with both feet on the floor and ground yourself by imagining that huge, thick roots are growing out of your body and lodging themselves deep in the earth.

2. Now, imagine a sphere of white light completely enveloping you, wrapping you in a protective cocoon of energy.

3. State your intention of wanting to open the chakras in your hands.

4. Slightly bend your fingers and bring the palms together, so they're nearly touching. Become aware of any sensations in your palms or in the space between them.

5. Slowly move your hands away from each other until they're about 15 centimetres (6 inches) apart.

6. Now, move them towards each other again, maintaining a slight gap between them, keeping them apart.

7. Move your hands together and apart again, keeping them further away from each other this time, always ensuring that your palms are facing each other.

8. Repeat this exercise until you can sense the energy building up between your palms. It will feel bouncy and elastic, like a soft rubber ball. You may also notice that the palms of your hands are tingling or it may feel as though a circle of energy has opened up in each one. This tells you that your hand chakras are open.

9. Once you've finished, imagine the chakras in your hands closing down and then remember to wash your hands, to cleanse them of any residual energy and to end the exercise.

Assessing and Healing Someone's Energy Field

1. Find a time when you, and the person whose energy you'll be scanning, are both relaxed and won't be disturbed. Switch off your phones, if you carry them. Ask the other person (the 'friend') to lie down on a bed or sofa, and make sure that they're comfortable and warm enough.

2. First, ask silent permission to tune in to your friend's energy field, because this is their sacred space. Tune in to them by holding their feet firmly but gently, to pick up their vibration.

3. Keeping your palms about 10 to 12 centimetres (4 to 5 inches) above your friend's body, use your hands to scan their energy field. Work up and down the area above their arms, legs, torso and head to check for any energy blockages. These will be areas of a different texture. They may feel hot or cold, prickly, dense or woolly.

4. Begin by concentrating on healing what's out of balance at a spiritual level – known as soul wounds.

5. Choose an oil that has an affinity with the sensations you're detecting (for example, Violet Leaf for extreme grief). Shake a couple of drops of the oil onto the palm of your hand, then move your hand around the person's body, always keeping it about 16 centimetres (6 inches) away from them. Remember, you're scanning the energy around them – you're not touching them physically.

6. If you need confirmation that a specific area is blocked, you can use an energy chime bar or a singing bowl to show you exactly where the blockage is. Sound the chime or bowl, sweeping it over the body. You'll hear the tone dip when it encounters the blockage. Hovering above the blockage with the note toning and a few drops of oil on the palms of your hands is often enough to release the energy and ease the soul wound. Consciously release the blockage, allowing the energy to flow once again.

Once the flow of energy is restored, the friend having the treatment usually feels much calmer and steadier. Above all when doing this work, the myrrhophore must be a good, active listener, hearing not only what the friend is saying, but also that which is unspoken. The friend may need to talk about or review their life, and they may also seek to find meaning in life events. The myrrhophore can help here through listening and asking gentle guiding questions or by offering insight from a place of non-judgement.

If the friend desires, the myrrhophore can help in working with spirit helpers, ancestors or other beings to promote soul healing. Guides, ancestors or helpers from the spirit world are often called in to assist during a sacred treatment. In shamanic work, these discarnate helpers have always been honoured as the connection between the spirit realms and us. During a healing with an oil, we might call on their help to heal aspects of the soul, the nature of which may be beyond our limited human understanding. These beings see the bigger picture of the cosmos, while we only see from our limited earthly perspective. They may be silently called upon to help at the beginning of a meditation or healing session and thanked at the end for their intervention.

Healing Soul Wounds

We all have soul wounds – deep places of pain and hurt that shape our lives to some extent. Sometimes they come from a traumatic event in childhood or they may come from abusive relationships and situations, toxic relationships with others (and ourselves) and addictions. They may also follow us from a past life or might be absorbed by us through our ancestral line. Typical soul wounds include:

◊   Feeling betrayed

◊   Feeling that we're not good enough

◊   Feeling that we've been abandoned

◊   Feeling that we've been born into the wrong body

◊   Feeling like an outsider

◊   Extreme grief

◊   Separation from twin souls/sacred partners

As explained earlier, sacred oils can help to heal soul wounds.

Anointing

Anointing, in which a sacred oil is smeared onto a part of the body, can be defined as a ritualized blessing. Anointing someone is a very sacred and devotional act. It's another service performed by myrrhophores to soothe the soul and spirit, and to mark certain rites of passage. A sacred ritual since time immemorial, it's common to many religions and belief systems, bringing both physical and spiritual benefits. The act of pouring oil onto the body (often the head) is called unction. In religious terms, anointing is seen as a nurturing ritual to nourish and prepare the soul before it embarks on a sacred journey, which is why anointing (referred to as 'extreme unction'), especially in the Roman Catholic faith, is often performed on the dying and the dead.

Priests and myrrhophores anoint a person to symbolize that something within them has been released. When we anoint someone who's undergoing any kind of transition, we can focus on releasing emotional blocks such as guilt and fear, as well as shedding unhelpful beliefs. Myrrhophores and soul midwives anoint the sick and dying with a sacred anointing oil, made by filling a dark glass bottle with 10ml of organic rapeseed oil and then adding the following three oils:

1. Rose oil: three drops

2. Frankincense oil: three drops

3. Sandalwood oil: three drops

Before anointing someone, you must prepare yourself by meditating and clearing your mind. Make sure that you're fully grounded and fully present in the moment. Blend your chosen sacred oil with some organic rapeseed oil. Before you begin the anointing process, remember to use your favourite method of psychic protection, such as imagining that a bubble of light surrounds your entire body, giving you total protection.

When you're ready, dip your thumb in the sacred oil, then place it on the forehead (the third eye) of the person you're working with. State the intention of the anointing act. For instance, you might say, 'I anoint you, Sarah-Jane, to witness that your fear of heights might be released and trouble you no longer.'

Coming Back into Balance

Learning to bring ourselves back into balance is essential after working with the intense energies of the oils. We can do this by:

1. Grounding and centring ourselves. Any physical activity can help here, such as walking, swimming or exercising in the gym. It's also good to eat foods with healthy carbohydrates, because these are very grounding.

2. Cleansing our energy fields so they're sparkly clean (*see Cleansing the Aura with Essential Oils, page 55*).

3. Closing our chakras to stop our energy from leaking out. Visualize your chakras, which spin horizontally throughout the body. (They look like CD discs spinning in a straight column that runs through the centre of the body.) When we meditate or are involved in sacred work, our chakras open

wide like lotus blossoms. After we've finished, we need to remember to close our chakras again, so that their petals are tightly closed. We can do this by imagining the petals of each chakra folding tight, chakra by chakra, beginning at the base and working up to the crown chakra.

4. Re-energizing our fields to help them to come back into balance. Drinking water, clapping your hands, dancing on the spot, doing some drumming or smelling some Fragonia oil will help to bring you back into balance once more.

5. Replenishing our reserves of energy so that we aren't running on empty. We can do this by getting enough sleep, eating small nutritious meals, drinking plenty of water, spending as much time as possible outside in the fresh air and doing things that bring us joy, such as being with our loved ones.

Soul Loss

Although soul loss is recognized in shamanic practice, it isn't as well known in other healing modalities. When we've worked with sacred oils to help another person, we may be vulnerable to soul loss if we've journeyed into other dimensions. Soul loss happens when we've unconsciously left a part of ourselves behind in another place and not grounded ourselves properly on our return.

We're usually protected from this happening simply by being mindful of the need to call in all parts of ourselves after working with the oils. This is why it's so important to ground ourselves after working with the oils, ensuring that we're fully present in our body again. We can ground ourselves by walking barefoot outside, shaking our hands and feet, imagining roots growing from us deep into the earth, and eating a high-carbohydrate meal.

Keeping Safe

After sacred work, especially when facilitating transition, you'll have generated a great deal of energy. Try not to hug or touch people until you've sealed your aura and restored your balance again (*see page 53*).

Cleansing the Aura with Essential Oils

We collect a lot more than dust and dirt on our feet. We also accumulate a lot of energy from the places where we walk and we need to rid ourselves of it on a regular basis. In addition, we release most of our energy through our lower legs and feet. This is why Jesus washed the disciples' feet – he was washing off more than just the day's grime.

Keeping our lower legs and feet clean at an energetic level helps to revitalize us, because it means our energy can flow freely again. This enables us to be more effective healers.

To make a cleansing mixture, add a few drops of Palo Santo to a bowl of warm water. Stir the mixture and pour a little onto your hands, then rub your hands together as though you're washing them. Now, use this mixture to wash your feet and lower legs. It will release the negative energy that's accumulated on your body, helping you to attract positive energy instead.

Psychopomp Work

A psychopomp is an experienced practitioner who accompanies the dead for part of the way on their last journey. This may involve being physically present when somebody dies, helping them to cross over right there and then. Psychopomp shamans have the skill to accompany a dying person with their spirit body, in order to show them the way into the beyond.

Most of the time, the psychopomp will be called to help the spirits of those who are trapped in the lower astral regions or who have become earthbound in what's called the Middle World, which is the astral side of our physical reality. Even though their physical bodies have gone, their energy bodies may still linger here, although they're not supposed to. Instead of moving on or 'going into the light', many spirits become earthbound. There are various reasons for that, such as guilt, fear, religious conditioning, unfinished business or lack of spiritual energy to move to the higher planes. Excessive grief experienced by the loved ones who are left behind, and their inability to let go of the person who's died, can also cause a spirit to become earthbound.

Unfortunately, these spirits usually don't know how to move on and may get stuck permanently or until somebody comes to their rescue. Here, the psychopomp shaman can help.

Galbanum is the sacred oil used for psychopomp work. However, this is very serious work, and shouldn't be performed without lengthy and proper training. This is because it involves opening ourselves up to unknown and possibly negative energies.

Practical Matters

Sacred oils must be treated with respect at all times, because they're energetic forces and spiritual entities. The more you work with them, the greater your understanding and appreciation of them will be, and the stronger your relationship with them will become.

Buying Oils

You should only buy the best sacred oils you can afford. You'll be asking them to do such important and powerful work that they need to be of the highest quality; otherwise, they'll disappoint you. Oils that are organic (cultivated, grown and harvested without chemicals) or wildcrafted (grown in the wild without human intervention and harvested with care) are best. There's a list of recommended suppliers at the back of the book (*see page 249*).

Storage

Make sure you store your oil blends away from heat and moisture. Keep them in dark-coloured glass bottles, which you can buy online, and be sure to label each one. Write the date on the label and use within six months.

Blending

I use organic rapeseed oil as the base for the sacred oils, because it's thick and it holds the vibration of the oils very well. Whenever you mix an oil, it's important to ensure you're in the right frame of mind, because the oil will absorb the energies you're transmitting. I never work with the oils when I feel out of sorts. Instead, I wait until I'm in a good mood and I often play a suitable piece of music while I work. I never use more than one sacred oil at a time when I'm using them therapeutically, unless I'm mixing a special oil for anointing (*see page 51*).

Safety

The quantities of essential oils used in sacred work are very small and they're always blended in a carrier oil, but you still need to take care when working with them. Essential oils are highly concentrated substances and should be treated with great respect. Some constituents of essential oils may be toxic, especially when used on the elderly, young people and pregnant women.

Certain oils may cause allergic reactions in sensitive people. Always carry out a skin test before using an essential oil, especially if you suffer from hay fever or other allergies. To do this, put a drop of the oil on a small piece of cotton wool and place on the skin on the back of the wrist or the inside of the elbow. Tie a piece of fabric around it to hold the cotton wool in place and leave for 24 hours, then remove it and examine the skin to see if it shows a reaction. If it does, the person is allergic to that particular oil and shouldn't use it.

Remember these important points:

1. Always dilute the essential oil in a carrier oil before applying it to the skin.

2. Follow the supplier's recommended dosages and dilutions.

3. Avoid using the oils on children under the age of three without prior consultation from a qualified aromatherapist.

4. Dilutions for children and the elderly should be at least half the recommended adult dose. Always seek professional advice if you're uncertain about what to do.

5. Always keep the oils out of reach of children and pets.

6. Keep oils away from the eyes.

7. Always store oils in a dark cupboard away from direct sunlight.

8. Never take oils internally unless you've been professionally advised to do so.

9. If you have epilepsy, high blood pressure or any other medical condition, seek the advice of a professional aromatherapist or medical practitioner before using an essential oil.

Using Oils During Pregnancy

Oils should always be used with caution during pregnancy. The essential oils in this book that should be completely avoided during pregnancy are:

◊ Cedarwood Atlas

◊ Galbanum

◊ Holy Basil

◊ Marigold

◊ Myrrh

◊ Myrtle

◊ Ravensara

◊ Rose Otto

◊ Yarrow

Also Remember...

Pure oils, whether they're organic or wildcrafted, are becoming increasingly difficult to source. I often wait months for a tiny 1ml bottle of aromatic oil to arrive in the post from a far-flung location such as the Amazon, India or even a remote village in France.

Sacred oils can be very expensive. Elecampane, which is one of the most precious sacred oils, has a global market price set at about £420 (US$550) an ounce and cannabis flower oil, which helps to dissolve both soul and physical pain, has a market price of over £700 (US$920) at the time of writing. One of my suppliers is a small family living in India with one solitary oil-producing tree growing on their land. From this, they harvest just 900ml or so of essential oil a year. The sales from this are their main source of income.

Another supplier of Violet oil is an elderly lady in France. She distils tiny quantities in an old copper still that's been in her family for generations. Her minuscule harvest fills about half an eggcup each spring. It's oil is sublime and helps countless people who are coping with extreme grief, so its value is truly beyond money. However, EU regulations covering the sale of such products make it impossible for her to sell her precious wares to the public, because her harvest is economically unviable. I now make my own Violet oil, but on a tiny and very painstaking scale.

The scarcity and expense of some oils means that many inferior and adulterated oils are now flooding the market. If an oil looks too cheap to be true, then it probably is. Nevertheless, not all of these sacred oils are expensive and they're available to most of us, bringing us riches for the heart and soul for the price of a pizza. I recently bought a bottle of excellent lavender oil from a high street chain for a mere £1 (US$1.30).

Exotic, fragrant, aromatic, rare and precious, sacred oils are medicines for both the soul and spirit. Gentle but powerful, sacred and profound, they work with us at the deepest level, bringing healing and expanding consciousness.

I hope that my exploration into the deep and esoteric world of sacred oils inspires your own journey. If we can nurture the profound sanctuary within, we can become the luminous beings that we're designed to be, truly engaging with our spiritual destiny.

The ancients, with their mystical knowledge, knew that human evolution and ascension always come from within and from the soul. They also understood the multidimensional universe that we inhabit, and were easy and confident travellers across the realms.

Sacred oils are the keys that open the doors to our inner consciousness, the seat of the soul and other dimensions. For those who 'know' and have 'eyes to see', this is why sacred oils are so extraordinary, elusive and fragile. These oils are as important in our modern, unsettled times as they were thousands of years ago, and they're as potent as ever.

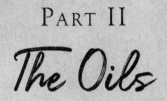

PART II

The Oils

Angelica

A Master Teacher

*'It is one of the gifts of great spiritual teachers to make
things simple. It is one of the gifts of their followers to
complicate them again. Often we need to scrape away
the accumulated complications of a master's message
in order to hear the kernel of what they said.'*

JULIA CAMERON,
GOD IS NO LAUGHING MATTER

Angelica is one of my personal totem oils. It's an exquisite oil with an extremely high vibration, with a reputation for attuning us to information already known to our higher self and even to knowledge passed down from previous lifetimes.

This oil is welcoming, has a gentle energy and is easy to connect with. It encourages us to ask questions, yet it won't try to sway our growth by giving us direct answers. It guides us thoughtfully, often imparting unexpected and surprising insights.

Botanical Information

There are about 60 species of Angelica, but Angelica oil is steam distilled from *Angelica archangelica*. This stately plant, which is native to Europe and parts of Asia, grows up to 2.5 metres (8 feet) tall. Its thick and hairy stems (which are traditionally candied and used as a culinary decoration), deeply divided leaves and large umbels of flowers make a dramatic architectural statement. It's often short-lived, despite being a hardy perennial, but it's a prolific self-seeder.

Angelica oil is distilled either from Angelica roots or seeds. The former produces a colourless oil that turns yellow with age and has an earthy scent. Oil distilled from the seeds is colourless and has a spicy aroma.

Angelica's Legendary Power

As you can tell from its name, this oil has a very strong connection with the angelic realms, especially with Archangel Michael, who's known for being the toughest of all spiritual warriors, as well as a teacher of divine truths.

He offers psychic protection to all who ask for it and is a 'don't mess with me' type of angel. In Angelica oil, his pure, fierce energy is distilled into an aromatic substance. Although refined and sophisticated, Angelica oil offers tough love and expects us to pull our weight as part of the healing dynamic.

In times past, the oil had the reputation for warding off the evil eye, and also for lifting spells and curses. It shields us against dark forces. In addition, Angelica is linked with the Holy Ghost.

Carmelite water, which is made by boiling Angelica roots, is said to have been invented in 1611 by Carmelite monks in Paris. It was made as a tonic for strength and protection against evil forces.

Another story claims that in 1665, an angel told an English monk in a dream that Angelica would cure the plague (which struck England that same year, killing thousands of people). Angelica subsequently became a chief ingredient in an official remedy called 'The King's Majesty's excellent remedy for the plague'. It was grown around monasteries and was referred to as 'angel grass'.

Angelica's Esoteric Qualities

Angelica's links with the angels means that it bestows on us their power and protection. It strengthens our aura, thereby increasing our ability to attune to the Divine and the spirit world, while also being able to connect with the material world around us. This makes it an invaluable oil when performing healing work, because it provides protection against negative energies, emotions and situations.

Angelica has the ability to transmute high angelic power, so that it will match our dense human vibration. It also aligns with certain humans, so they can take on the role of 'earth angels', administering protective powers to others who are struggling with fear or trauma. Angelica's presence is huge, bringing with it courage and love, with its very exalted angelic energy.

If we're undergoing a shamanic journey for ourselves, this can sometimes feel like a 'trial of madness'. Angelica holds us safe while we absorb the experience.

When to Use Angelica

We can call on the spirit of Angelica oil for courage, strength and help in any situation. If you're visiting anywhere with negative energy, Angelica will take care of you. But you must remember to ask it for help; otherwise you won't receive it.

Angelica's protective qualities are also very helpful for anyone who feels under psychic attack and is trying to cope or for when they're recovering from the effects of a psychic attack. In addition, it offers good protection against energy vampires – those who drain our energy until we feel exhausted and they're thriving. If you need clarity in order to look into the hearts of others, Angelica will provide it.

You can use Angelica when performing rituals in which you cut the energetic cords that bind you to toxic people or difficult situations. It's also excellent as part of your energetic toolbox when releasing attachments and spirit entities.

Karmic Roots

As its name suggests, Angelica has karmic links with the angels.

According to St Thomas Aquinas, who was inspired by the writings of Pseudo-Dionysius the Areopagite, the angelic realms consist of nine choirs of angels, each of which has a specific role:

◊ Seraphim guard God's throne

◊ Cherubim have perfect knowledge

◊ Thrones enact God's decisions

◊ Dominions manifest the glory of God

◊ Virtues create miracles and give courage to humans

◊ Powers fight the forces of evil

◊ Principalities protect the world's religions

◊ Archangels are the link between God and humans

◊ Angels work directly with humans

Guided Meditation

You might like to record this meditation before meditating with Angelica oil. This will enable you to relax and listen to the meditation without unnecessary distractions. Simply follow the instructions for preparing yourself for a guided meditation (*see page 35*).

> *I'm the 'divine' teacher of teachers, making a bridge between the visible and invisible worlds. My presence opens a doorway between body and spirit.*
>
> *In order to heal the body, we must heal the spirit and bathe it in light, repairing any tears and holes that have let in the darkness.*
>
> *I can show you the psychic causes of illness intuitively or in mythical dream language. I'll encourage you to work with passion and purpose, to travel wisely with courage, inspired and strengthened by the light in your heart.*
>
> *Use me in sacred rites, to seek growth and value in your life. You'll see a vision of the 'whole' when travelling through uncharted territories of spirit. You'll realize that wise thoughts and skills will break the rigid bonds of living with fear and uncertainty, so you can birth your inner power into the light.*

Angelica's Key Points

◊ Connected with Archangel Michael

◊ Helps us to move into a higher consciousness

◊ Opens our hearts

◊ Protects from negative energies and emotions

◊ Scent – earthy or spicy

◊ Affinity with the heart chakra

Contraindications

◊ The oil made from Angelica seeds has fewer contraindications than the oil made from the roots.

◊ Both versions of Angelica are emmenagogues (they can induce or help menstruation), so shouldn't be used during pregnancy.

◊ Both versions of Angelica can be phototoxic (they react to ultraviolet light, causing possible blistering and inflammation of the skin), so should not be applied directly to the skin.

◊ Neither version should be used if you're diabetic.

CASE STUDY

Ava is a young woman who's starting out as a very gifted healer. Her reputation for quickly seeing 'dis-ease' and healing brings many people to her busy clinic.

However, she was beginning to feel increasingly toxic and heart-weary. Ava was giving so much of herself in her work that she felt as if her clients were transferring their illnesses onto her. She also sensed dark, 'life-sucking' energy forms around her, like spirit attachments. Ava didn't know how to cope and even considered having to give up her work:

'I was feeling very alone, lost and discouraged. I couldn't ignore the feelings of unrest inside me. They brought a sense of spiritual crisis. I was on the edge and I felt as though I were falling apart and dissolving.

'At the end of one long day when I'd seen eight clients, I felt I'd reached a crossroads. I knew that I couldn't go on as I was.

'I sat down, sobbing and exhausted, and simply asked for help. After some time, a silence seemed to descend and then a rush of wind filled the room. In my mind's eye, I could see a flash of blue and a force field weaving in and out, around my body. From nowhere, hands were placed on my shoulders, and I was filled with a feeling of sweetness and calm. I asked, "Who are you?" and the name "Michael" came to me. I knew exactly who this angelic force was.

'Without words, Archangel Michael told me that I was free of all entities and energies, and that a field of protection would surround me from now on. All I ever needed was to call and ask for help, and it would come.

'Later, I remembered I had a bottle of Angelica essential oil on the shelf in my bedroom. I removed the top and inhaled the aroma. It matched the energy I'd felt when Archangel Michael visited me.

A symbol came into my mind and I quickly scribbled it down, knowing he'd sent it to me as a sign.

'I now use Angelica oil to paint a protective symbol, using my finger, on the door of my treatment room before patients arrive. It helps to keep me pristine, as well as to work without absorbing other people's energies, emotions and illnesses.

'When I connect with Archangel Michael, his energy feels warm and loving. He has a fiery spirit and will greet you with unconditional love, regardless of your current circumstances. He also taught me how to look after myself.'

Cedarwood Atlas

Strength of Spirit

'Those who are steadfastly balanced, humble, and in harmony with the Sage inherit everything under the sun.'
TA YU/POSSESSION IN GREAT MEASURE, *I CHING*

Cedarwood Atlas oil has been revered for its spicy, warm and woody scent since ancient times. It's been used to make incense as well as essential oil, and the fragrant cedarwood itself has been used to construct temples and palaces.

This is a very warming and strengthening oil. If you feel afraid and burdened with anxiety, Cedarwood Atlas oil is wonderful for bringing you courage and strength. It helps you to feel strong, supported and optimistic about the outcome of any situation you're facing, giving you an extra boost when needed.

Botanical Information

Many different oils go by the name 'Cedarwood' and each has its own properties. However, some aren't made from cedarwood at all, despite their names. For instance, Texas Cedarwood and Virginian Cedarwood are both made from juniper trees.

Cedarwood Atlas oil is made from the Atlantic cedar (*Cedrus atlantica*), which is a stately evergreen tree that grows up to 40 metres (130 feet) tall. The wood is hard and highly aromatic, because it contains such a high percentage of essential oil. The oil is extracted from wood chips using steam distillation. It ranges in colour from yellow to amber.

Cedarwood Atlas's Legendary Power

The word 'cedar' comes from the Semitic word for 'power'. Cedar is known as the tree of life, and is a renowned symbol of strength and faith. Cedarwood Atlas has been honoured for its meditative and relaxing qualities since ancient times. Its ceremonial use alone was recorded over 2,000 years ago.

Incense made from Cedarwood Atlas was sacred to the ancients. The wood was used by King Solomon to build his glorious temple, as described in Kings 1:5-7.

The trade in Cedarwood Atlas was mentioned on a clay tablet dating from 1800BCE. The Egyptians used Cedarwood Atlas oil for mummification and other funerary rites. They also believed that it extended life and helped to give immortality.

Cedarwood Atlas's Esoteric Qualities

In the myrrhophore tradition, Cedarwood Atlas is often used by a priestess when she prepares for initiations. Traditionally, this might have involved being locked in a small cave in the dark for several days, working with snakes and other wild animals in order to increase her energy skills. Myrrhophores might also do some astral travelling in order to source information for someone they're healing. When the journey ahead is going to be demanding (and possibly terrifying), you can call on Cedarwood Atlas for its calm, peaceful and strengthening presence.

I often wear a Cedarwood Atlas mala (a string of prayer beads), made and blessed by Buddhist nuns, to strengthen my energy field, especially when I've been working with very sick people in hospices.

When to Use Cedarwood Atlas

Himalayan Cedarwood Atlas is one of the most spiritually and emotionally grounding essential oils of all. It's used by Tibetan Buddhists as temple incense. Being grounded is an essential skill for healers; otherwise, the emotions that they intuitively pick up from both the people and the environment around them could easily affect them. This can knock them off balance, making them feel vulnerable and eventually even undermining their health.

When we're grounded, we're present in our body and connected with the Earth, allowing us to feel centred and balanced, no matter what's going on around us. This is why Cedarwood Atlas is so useful when preparing to do sacred work of any kind. It anchors us both in ourselves and in the here and now.

Cedarwood Atlas is also helpful for facing up to and letting go of difficult situations or relationships, especially when we feel they're holding us back. It can help us to release negativity in whichever form we experience it.

Karmic Roots

Cedarwood Atlas has karmic links with the Earth and with the elemental realms.

The Earth

In traditional astrology, the meaning of the Earth tends to be overlooked in favour of concentrating on the other planets in our solar system. Yet, to esoteric astrologers, the Earth has much to teach us. Our time on Earth is one in which we can learn, develop and be of service to others. At the same time, we're taking an inner journey in which we discover what we've come here to accomplish and how we'll be able to do it. In esoteric astrology, the Earth is the ruling planet of Sagittarius.

The Elemental Realms

Elementals are nature spirits – the creatures that populate fairy tales and children's books but are frequently dismissed by adults as being imaginary. Yet they're not. They exist, just as we do, and are an essential part of the life force of nature; without them, nothing on our planet would exist. Elementals include the salamanders of the fire element; gnomes of the earth element; sylphs of the air element; and undines of the water element. Fairies and elves are also members of the elemental kingdom.

Guided Meditation

You might like to record this meditation before meditating with Cedarwood Atlas. This will enable you to relax and listen to the meditation without unnecessary distractions. Simply follow the instructions for preparing yourself for a guided meditation (*see page 35*).

Visualize the immense power of the solid Cedarwood Atlas tree standing tall and know that this is a time of great power for you to access your own strength. I can help you to offer a powerful connection to your own higher self and divinity, and to the higher dimensions. I'm a powerful guide who can hold you through difficult times and support you whenever you need to stand in your own sovereignty.

We're all being called to step out of our old ways of being and to heal our core wounds. This takes courage and vision. I hold the boundary between the physical and the etheric planes, which is why I offer you the most powerful way to access your own seat of strength. This, you must summon from the essence of yourself that resides still in the spirit world.

I'm the messenger of the invisible world. Forget all your fears and let them go.

Cedarwood Atlas's Key Points

◊ Helps us to find our power and strength

◊ Fosters optimism and hope

◊ Helps to ground and anchor us

◊ Releases negative thoughts and emotions

◊ Scent – warm and woody

◊ Affinity with the base chakra

Contraindications

◊ Cedarwood Atlas is an abortifacient (able to induce an

abortion) and also an emmenagogue (able to help or induce menstruation), so should be completely avoided during pregnancy.

◊ It can cause local skin irritation for sensitive individuals, so should only be used when diluted in a carrier oil.

◊ Cedarwood Atlas oil can cause nausea when ingested, so should never be taken internally.

CASE STUDY

Talented opera singer Priti was signed up to do an exciting and important tour across the USA. However, she was now dreading the trip and was even thinking of cancelling it. She explained:

'I feel as though someone pulls my power from me just as I step on the stage. I can keep going up to a point, but the strength of my performance starts to tail off after 10 minutes or so. It's as if my inner battery goes flat.'

I asked Priti to lie on the floor, gave her a pillow and covered her with a blanket. I used a shamanic rattle to clear energy in the corners of the room and then in her body, from head to toe. Offering prayers for her, I then set the intention to 'see' what was happening to Priti every time she stepped out on stage. I found myself travelling back with her to when she was 20 years old, training to be an opera singer at a music academy. She was in a class with two other young women.

As the journey began, I shape-shifted into a Cedarwood Atlas tree.
I slipped inside the trunk, into its blackness, and searched for a
chink of light in the darkness. While travelling down to the roots of
the tree, I tapped into its deep wisdom to receive the information
that I needed about Priti.

From inside the tree, I watched the singing lesson. Priti was
praised lavishly by her singing teacher, who told her, in front of
the other students, that she had huge potential. If she worked hard
enough, she could easily be one of the top soloists of her generation.

The student standing next to her was so consumed with jealousy
that she uttered a curse. 'Yes, she might get on stage, but her voice
will desert her,' she muttered, half to herself. I believed this curse to
be at the core of Priti's problem.

We don't realize the power of our words. Wishes and curses are
as real now as they were in the fairy tales of the past. Curse-
banishing was once the stock-in-trade work of the wise women, yet
contemporary curses are just as potent.

Priti and I spent several weeks working with various oils, creating
an intention to bring her back into her full power, both on stage and
in her daily life. Cedarwood Atlas was one of those oils, and it both
increased and strengthened Priti's vibration. Once again she felt whole
and strong, completing her concert tour, which was a glorious success.

. . . .

Elemi

Letting Go, Surrender

'Our Father, which art in heaven,
Hallowed be thy name.
Thy kingdom come.
Thy will be done, on Earth as it is in Heaven.'
THE LORD'S PRAYER, MATTHEW 6:9–10

Each sacred oil has an energetic code that must be deciphered before we can gain access to deeper levels of understanding of how it can be used. Elemi has a particularly rich history and is one of the six oils that I always carry when working as a soul midwife, the others being Fragonia, Palo Santo, Ravensara, Rose and Spikenard. I also use it when holding vigil in the final days of someone's life, because it's so valuable in helping people to let go of this life and surrender to the next.

Botanical Information

Elemi is made from the resin and bark of *Canarium luzonicum*, which is a tropical tree that grows up to 30 metres (98 feet) tall and is native to the Philippines. It bears pale yellow leaves and when these sprout, the tree produces an exotic, honey-like, aromatic oleoresin. This solidifies when it comes into contact with the air, and the tree stops producing it when the last leaf falls at the end of the growing season. The oil is steam distilled and has a golden colour, with a pleasant, rich aroma that has hints of balsam, pine and lemon.

Elemi's Legendary Power

Elemi is a traditional Arabic oil whose names translates as 'heaven and Earth'. It was used in the Middle East, and later throughout Europe, to make medicines and incense, in addition to perfume, soaps and creams. Elemi was used extensively in ancient Egypt in part of the embalming process. It's believed to have strengthened the connection between the deceased and their ancestral lineage. It also ensures that the link between them remains strong and unbreakable, helping the soul in its onward journey through the underworld. This is another clue to Elemi's sacred properties and another connection with its meaning of 'heaven and Earth'. It reminds us that the sacred resin in the tree supports our wellbeing on both the spiritual and physical planes.

In ancient times, sacred essential oils were regarded as a source of power and divination. They were used to anoint kings, cure sickness, and provide the magic and power in rituals and ceremonies, but knowledge of them was strictly confined to those who knew how to work with them. Elemi was one of the best-kept secrets of all, enabling a swift and joyous passage from one realm to another, and certainly between heaven and Earth, as well as also into more mysterious faery realms.

Elemi's Esoteric Qualities

Smelling this oil – even holding the bottle while tuning in to Elemi's exquisite golden energy – is like holding a bottle of spinning gold. The energy feels as though it's dancing and soaring. Elemi is a conduit for accessing the ecstatic energies of the Divine.

Its delicate, spicy, warm and slightly honey-tinged aroma belies its complex matrix. To the inexperienced user, it may give a sensation of sweetness and gentle comfort. But as you delve deeper, with intention, Elemi may reveal herself as a noble and heightened teacher of cosmic ecstasy.

When to Use Elemi

Soul midwives often use this oil when someone is very close to death but appears to be hesitant and anxious about surrendering to the process, even though the time has come for them to leave this life. Elemi coaxes them into taking the leap and stepping into the unknown. It shows 'the way across the threshold', and also helps to remove doubts and fears in anyone with a phobia about dying. It's an oil of exquisite gentleness, coupled with the power of a golden laser, enabling swift and delicate transitions.

Elemi is an oil that helps people to make other major transitions in their life with ease and grace, too, whether it's moving from one house to another, emigrating to another country, starting a new relationship or beginning a new career. If you're standing at a major crossroads in life, you can use this oil to encourage and strengthen your soul, using any of the techniques described in Part I. Elemi enables you to trust that all is well and that a higher power is guiding you.

Karmic Roots

Elemi is connected with the Pleiades and Lemuria.

The Pleiades

Also known as the Seven Sisters, the Pleiades are an open cluster of between 300 and 500 stars in the constellation Taurus. Energy from the Pleiades is vibrant and uplifting, feminine and nurturing. In numerology, the number seven is connected with the thinker in search of truth. It also carries the archetype of the loner within. Linking this with the gentle guidance of Elemi and the influence of the Pleiades, we can glimpse, with deeper understanding, the individual quest to connect heaven with Earth.

Lemuria

Lemuria preceded Atlantis at the beginning of time. Whether or not it was an actual place on earth or a realm of consciousness is unknown. But it was a time before humans were given bodies, when they were beings of light and energy, with extreme sensitivity and an affinity with plants.

Lemurians were a highly evolved race, with strong spiritual beliefs and telepathic communications between both each other and all other life forms, including animals, water, plants and beings from other universes.

Guided Meditation

You might like to record this meditation before meditating with Elemi. This will enable you to relax and listen to the meditation without unnecessary distractions. Simply follow the instructions for preparing yourself for a guided meditation (*see page 35*).

My name weaves together heaven and Earth. I'm the silver cord or the ladder of gold that connects this world to the next. I'm the umbilical link between Mother Earth and Father Sky. I show the way for the soul and spirit.

Use me to lead you with total joy and trust to the light. I'll help you to hear your loved ones' voices welcoming you home from the other side. Allow me to escort you across the sacred threshold. I'll surround you with a cocoon of love and hope and joy. I'm your earthly connection with heaven, your passport to Paradise.

Elemi's Key Points

◊   Enables the transformation of consciousness

◊   Removes the fear of death during the dying process

◊   Used for embalming in ancient Egypt

◊   Supports all major life transitions

◊   Scent – warm, spicy, balsam, pine, lemon, slightly honeyed

◊   Affinity with the crown chakra

Contraindications

Don't work with Elemi if you're using any recreational drugs, because it may amplify their effects.

CASE STUDY

Joseph suffered from severe asthma and related heart disease. He had a deep fear of dying, which was partly caused by a haunting

anxiety about losing control, not only of his breath, but also of his bodily functions.

We worked together for nearly a year, exploring his underlying worries and concerns about his health. Joseph confided his fears in me:

'My fear of dying paralyses me when, during an asthma attack, I'm not able to breathe. All coping functions in my body close down. I'm just totally frozen in my body, holding on to myself. Even if someone's there to hold me, I'm alone in my struggle.

'This feels like my body and lungs and heart will explode. I'm on the edge of collapsing or fainting or wanting to faint, so I don't have to go through the experience. Better to pass out than go through not knowing whether I live or die. There's no way I can relax, meditate, breathe gently or even calm myself down. I have to ride through it all and hope for the best outcome.

'This can be a few minutes or, in some cases, as much as two hours. The embarrassing part is that when I'm in this state, my bowels want to open and I want to urinate, and of course this does happen and I have no say over it. My body takes over.

'I know this also happens when people are dying. Their functions just go. I've experienced this on hospital wards and late at night when having a big attack, wishing for death because of not wanting to go through what I was going through. And thinking *that, actually, death would be easier than trying to come out of an asthma attack.*

'Because, these days, my breathing is bad every day, I guess I visit near-death every day. Or my lungs can or could just give up. Or, as my chest consultant says, under the pressure of an attack, my heart will just go POP!

'I have real fear here as I've no control, none at all. I'm not in charge of my lungs or my body. Fear just takes over.'

Usually, soul midwives don't apply a sacred oil directly to a patient's skin. Instead, we apply it to our own hands and transfer the oil's energy by touch or by stroking it through the aura of the patient. But when working with Joseph, in one of our last sessions together, we talked about the idea of anointing as a rite of passage or blessing to release unhelpful fears. Joseph asked to be anointed on his crown chakra (on the top of his head), to represent his intention to work through his final fears, and so that is what I did.

This is what he said afterwards:

'There was something about the act of anointing that brought a loosening and a sense of grace to a very stuck and traumatic situation. I felt something heavy and constricted lift, and it's as if the Sun has come out.'

We worked with Elemi until Joseph's unexpected death in his sleep some three months later. His partner later shared that he'd slipped away very peacefully, smiling and restful in his sleep after a day out visiting some beautiful gardens.

. . . .

Fragonia™

For Transitions of Every Kind

*'We meditate on that divine sun, the true knight of
the shining ones. May it illuminate our minds.'*
THE GAYATRI VERSE OF THE VEDAS (C. 5000BCE)

Once you've worked with Fragonia, you'll never want to be
without it. Its light and joyful energy lifts and energizes
the spirit, bringing a feeling of optimism and balance. It's a very
cheerful, sunny oil, with a beguiling simplicity and charm that
feels both innocent and childlike, taking people by surprise
when they sniff the oil. 'Oh, I like this one,' they say as they take
a deeper sniff. Its spirit is solar-bright.

Botanical Information

Fragonia (*Agonis fragrans*), commonly called the coarse tea tree,
only grows in parts of Western Australia. It's a small evergreen
shrub that reaches about 2.4 metres (8 feet) high and bears small

globular white flowers. It was traditionally grown commercially for the floristry industry because of the exquisite scent of its flowers. The essential oil is steam distilled from the plant's leaves and terminal branches.

Fragonia is a modern oil and has only been made since 2005. It's the only essential oil in production to carry a trademark, to ensure that all of the oil sold under its name conforms to a specific chemotype.

Fragonia's Legendary Power

Because it's so new, there are no legends associated with Fragonia. Nevertheless, it's a remarkable oil because of its very unusual chemical mix. It's the only oil known to have all of its chemical constituents in almost perfect balance: its oxides, monoterpenes and monoterpenoids form a ratio of 1:1:1. This configuration is known as the 'golden ratio' or 'golden proportion', hinting at the affinity of Fragonia with cosmic balance and harmony. The golden ratio is an important part of sacred geometry, which is the name given to the sacred codes that make up the design of everything we know to exist.

Fragonia's Esoteric Qualities

This oil has appeared at the right time. I believe it's manifested to help humankind adjust to the rise in vibration as the planet's consciousness evolves. It comes from the Sun and has links with Ra, the Sun god. Its luminous energy radiates from this oil, touching everything with light, and it has the gift of lifting everything around it.

When used esoterically, Fragonia brings everything subtly back into balance, making it the perfect oil for anyone experiencing any kind of change. Not only does it bring a feeling of safety and balance, but it also brings clarity to muddled thinking.

In soul midwifery, which is the holistic and spiritual care of the dying, Fragonia is our number-one oil. It does so many things to help the dying to cope with the changes happening at the physical, psychospiritual and emotional levels.

Fragonia oil brings calm and balance, in addition to a sense of optimism, whenever it's used. In fact, we jokingly call it 'gin and tonic in a bottle'. Not only does it revive the spirits of the seriously ill, but it also perks up the healers when they have been working at full pelt. This makes me wonder how we ever lived without it.

Perhaps because it's such a new oil, it brings with it a rush of fresh energy entirely in keeping with a 'new age' in working with the dying and also people undergoing other major transitions. Fragonia acts as a subtle catalyst for change by realigning us with our inner core, so we can receive our soul's wisdom, gently releasing blocked emotions while restoring balance and peace of mind in troubled situations. It holds us while we let go and trust that whatever changes are coming will be for our soul's development.

When to Use Fragonia

The main message Fragonia imparts is 'Don't worry, I'll see you through this crisis. Just stay with me and I'll look after you.' For this reason, Fragonia comes to the rescue for anyone facing uncertain times, whether it's moving house, relocating to another country to begin a new job, beginning or ending a relationship, taking the plunge with a new project or dealing with any other serious life-altering challenge. It's a wise ally that packs a powerful punch in a good way and it smells of sunshine.

Fragonia comes into its own during the dying process. During this time, many energetic shifts are taking place, where the dying person is switching their emphasis from being in their physical body to becoming a light-filled and spiritual being.

Something for healers to note is that the fragrance of this oil is usually very well tolerated by people undergoing chemotherapy. Other oils with distinct smells may make the patient feel nauseated.

Karmic Roots

Fragonia has karmic links with the lost land of Lemuria in the Pacific Ocean (*see page 87*).

Guided Meditation

You might like to record this meditation before meditating with Fragonia. This will enable you to relax and listen to the meditation without unnecessary distractions. Simply follow the instructions for preparing yourself for a guided meditation (*see page 35*).

Embrace me and I'll bring you calm. I'm the colour of amber. I ebb and flow, in and out with the tides like the breath in your body. With the qualities of spirit living in water, I'm here to heal and balance, and to restore you into equilibrium and a healing state where all can be well again.

Call on me when you're exhausted as a result of pain or fear or the constant worry of trying to keep going. I'm able to enhance your connection with your higher self and remind you of what you really know but have forgotten. I'll also help with feelings of instability and anxiety when you're trying to integrate your emotions.

I'm here to support you through any form of change. I bring a lightness and strength to every waking moment, and I'll assist you as you progress from one vibrational change to the next. I smell of the sweet honey warmth of the undiminishing Sun. I'm sweet. I sing and laugh with you. Receive my joy and my strength.

Fragonia's Key Points

◊ A powerful and strong plant intelligence that comes with a mission

◊ Lifts the spirits and boosts optimism

◊ Supportive through any type of transition

◊ Well tolerated by people receiving chemotherapy

◊ Scent – spicy, honeyed and lemon

◊ Affinity with the solar plexus chakra

Contraindications

None known.

CASE STUDY

Having moved house three times in the past year, Kelly was exhausted. She was now about to join her boyfriend, Simon, in Alaska, where he's a research scientist. Although she loved and wanted to be with him, she was fearful about moving so far away from her friends and family. Having heard about the ability of

Fragonia to help with transitions of all kinds, Kelly asked her massage therapist to add it to a base oil when she had a weekly massage to help with a back problem.

During the massage, Kelly saw beautiful colours, even though her eyes were closed. When she described them to Simon, he said that her description reminded him of how he imagined the Northern Lights might look. Kelly was intrigued and began to paint pictures, trying to capture the colours and shapes that she'd seen. Eventually, she became increasingly inspired to learn more about the Northern Lights and her curiosity led her to research everything she could about this extraordinary natural phenomenon that seemed to speak to her so vividly.

It was as if lights had come on inside her. She was bright and the dullness in her eyes had cleared. Now, she was more than ready for the changes that lay ahead. She still believes that Fragonia was responsible for this life-enhancing shift in attitude.

. . . .

Frankincense

Aligning Spirit and Soul with the Divine

*'Every cell in your body has a direct relationship with the
Creative Life Force and each cell is independently responding.
When you feel joy, all the circuits are open, so the Life Force
can be fully received. When you feel guilt, blame, fear or
anger, the circuits are hindered and the Life Force cannot
flow as effectively. Physical experience is about monitoring
those circuits and keeping them as open as possible. Your
cells know what to do; they are summoning the Energy.'*

ABRAHAM HICKS, *ASK AND IT IS GIVEN*

Frankincense was one of the most highly valued commodities
of the ancient world and it's still of huge benefit today. It
has many healing properties that can help us to deal with our
modern hectic and chaotic pace of life. It's often coupled with
Myrrh (*see page 135*), although the two oils have very different
personalities. Nevertheless, both Frankincense and Myrrh help
us to heal soul wounds.

Botanical Information

The oil, which can be pale yellow or slightly green, is steam distilled from the creamy white aromatic resin (oleoresin) harvested from trees of the Boswellia family. These are native to East and Central Africa, and also Ethiopia, Yemen, Oman, Saudi Arabia and Somalia. The trees are usually between 3 and 7 metres (10 and 22 feet) high. The scent of Frankincense oil is fresh and slightly citrusy, with floral rosy hints and balsamic woody notes.

Frankincense's Legendary Power

Frankincense's name is derived from '*franc*', meaning pure, and '*insensium*', meaning to smoke. We can understand from this that it was used to help to prepare a space (such as in a temple or church), and to purify the heart in readiness for prayer and meditation. It was, and still is, used in censers (also known as thuribles) by priests before performing their rites – the fumes were said to send the congregation into a state of ecstasy while saying their prayers.

Many civilizations, including the ancient Egyptians, Babylonians, Greeks, Persians and Romans, have valued Frankincense for its ritual and sacred properties. It was one of the three gifts brought by the Magi to Jesus's Nativity. The Magi were very astute in their choice of gifts, because each one was sacred and had esoteric powers. In the case of Frankincense, the gift was all about connection to spirit and the Divine – an extremely fitting present for a child destined to change the world.

Frankincense features in a Greek myth. In *Metamorphoses*, Ovid wrote that Helios, the Sun god, loved a mortal woman called Leucothoe. Her jealous father had her buried alive, but Helios warmed the ground that covered her and she was reborn as the Frankincense tree.

Frankincense's Esoteric Qualities

This oil helps to open the third eye in order to understand sacred wisdom and 'see' the gifts of spirit. It also strengthens our spiritual connections, as well as nurturing and supporting our growth during spiritual attainment.

Frankincense oil works on many complex levels, linking up and repairing broken energy threads that were created during past lives, which have linked us to people and places that are hampering our spiritual wellbeing. The oil repairs soul wounds that follow on from a past life and reappear in the current life, such as addictions and obsessions. It acts as a soothing balm, and is very healing for delicate and burned-out energy fields.

Traditional Chinese Medicine recognizes the importance of Frankincense, using it regulate the flow of qi (energy) through the body. This energy flows from the physical body out to the subtle energy fields, thereby recharging the aura.

Frankincense helps us to add spiritual awareness to the intellect by opening the intelligence contained within the heart. In esoteric terms, this is sometimes known as calling in the *nous* (*see page 15*). It has the power to attune us to Christ Consciousness, which is the merging of mind, body and spirit manifesting as God's love on Earth.

Meditating with Frankincense slows down the breathing and deepens the breath. When we're born, we come in on a breath, and when we die, we go out on a breath. Frankincense carries the mechanism of this energy. Breathing connects the astral and physical bodies, igniting the spark of spiritual life. Frankincense calms and soothes, steadies restlessness and helps the overactive mind. It also helps us to heal obsessive memories from the past.

Frankincense has so many spiritual properties that it could take a lifetime of serious study to reveal all of its potential.

When to Use Frankincense

Frankincense has many invaluable uses. It can help to clear away melancholy and also to ease the sadness that can be associated with nostalgic thoughts. It's a marvellous aid when dealing with any kind of spiritual crisis, because it not only soothes our inner chaos, but it also provides spiritual comfort and protection. We can use it to give spiritual direction whenever important decisions are needed and it can also help to dispel accidie, which is a form of spiritual drought in which we feel apathetic. Frankincense can even be used to consecrate a sacred space. Its ability to open the third eye makes it helpful in oneiromancy, which is divination using dreams.

Frankincense invites us to prepare to embrace our darkness – the parts of ourselves that we don't always feed with love and light. Introspection and the ability to explore our inner world are requirements for knowing our true, authentic selves.

In addition, this oil eases compulsive or obsessive behaviour, such as the uncontrollable desire for food, tobacco, drugs or alcohol. It calms the active mind and increases the self-esteem in order to better resist such cravings.

Karmic Roots

Frankincense has strong associations with the planet Saturn.

Before the development of telescopes, Saturn was the most distant planet visible with the naked eye. Its connection with Frankincense denotes the development of intuition, understanding and concentration, and the communication of universal law. In Roman mythology, Saturn was the equivalent of the Greek god Chronos, who governed time. Therefore, Saturn rules the wisdom and maturity that come with age.

In astrology, Saturn is the ruling planet of Capricorn and, before Uranus was discovered, of Aquarius. Saturn's lessons for us involve being grounded, realizing not only our strengths, but also our weaknesses, and learning from experience.

Key Points

◊   Soothes inner chaos

◊   Provides spiritual comfort

◊   Eases compulsive or obsessive behaviour

◊   Consecrates a sacred space

◊   Scent – earthy, with floral, rosy, balsamic notes

◊   Aligned with the brow and crown chakras

Contraindications

None known.

Guided Meditation

You might like to record this meditation before meditating with Frankincense. This will enable you to relax and listen to the meditation without unnecessary distractions. Simply follow the instructions for preparing yourself for a guided meditation (*see page 35*).

> *Breathe deeply, switch off your mind and slow down. Know that God is love and that love is harmony. These are both the highest*

aspects of the Divine. When life seems dry and difficult, it's often because the patterns in the holograph of your psychic memory are incomplete. I'll help you to reclaim the consciousness that may have been lost because of your disconnection from spirit. As you reconnect with spirit, new holographic patterns will emerge for you.

Use me to open your third eye to bring yourself inner vision, as well as to restore balance to the left and right sides of your brain. My energy is light and ethereal – as it passes between spirit and soul, this creates a sense of 'quickening'. I'll align your etheric, mental and causal bodies, transferring memories from other lifetimes back to you while you're in the dream state.

CASE STUDY

George was a young and very conscientious priest in charge of a large and demanding inner-city parish. He loved his work and devoted his time to working with many diverse groups – young adults, a women's refuge and a day centre for Alzheimer's patients – as well as offering spiritual care and companionship to his flock.

He gave of himself constantly and willingly, but noticed how fatigued he was becoming. He began to fear that he was running on empty, but it never occurred to him that he might cut back on his duties. George was no longer feeling any nourishment for his own soul and was increasingly disturbed by his sense of spiritual isolation.

George needed Frankincense. Although it has a gentle and soft energy, it's renowned for its ability to slice through apathy and awaken the inner senses. Ancient temple priests knew this, using it to amplify their power and enhance their own energy fields. George was familiar with Frankincense because he used it in his church, but he didn't understand its healing power and was curious to learn more.

We began with a simple guided meditation, in which George concentrated on the rhythm of his breathing, placing a few drops of Frankincense oil on his heart chakra. We lit a candle to keep George's focus soft.

His aura, which had looked dull and grey when he began the meditation, became brighter and clearer almost immediately. The colours surrounding his chakras rippled and merged into each other as his energy field rebalanced itself. This is often how the oils work, because they show clairvoyantly where harmony has been disrupted and energy has become stagnant. George breathed in deeply and began to expand his energy field. It was as though a muddy puddle was becoming clear again.

It took several weeks for George to become fully balanced again, but gradually his joy and inspiration returned. And so did his link with God. He also learned the lesson that many healers have to suffer before they can fully help others. Anyone whose job involves giving deeply of themselves must regularly receive some healing themselves or their reserves of energy will run dry.

. . . .

Galbanum

Opening Portals, Psychopomp

'It is important to know that every single human being, from the moment of birth until the moment when we make the transition and end this physical existence, is in the presence of guides or guardian angels who will wait for us and help us in the transition from life to life after death.'

ELISABETH KÜBLER-ROSS, *ON DEATH AND DYING*

Myrrhophores see working with the souls of the dead as a sacred part of their service. The name for this is psychopomp, which is an ancient Greek term for the conductor of souls. Psychopomps perform their work in many ways, through sacred ritual, channelling or sitting in a circle with others. They're also known as soul rescuers, pontiffs and shamans. As such, they work with the recently dead, lost souls who are searching for the light, as well as large groups of souls who have died after a catastrophic event, such as a tsunami or a battle.

Many psychopomps do their work quietly in hospitals, hospices and within the community. Some do this work openly, while others perform it during sleep and meditation without even being conscious of doing so.

This is deeply profound work and when done consciously, with intent, it's always performed with great reverence and compassion. Galbanum oil has a long history of assisting in soul ritual work and can help by forming a bridge across the sacred threshold.

Botanical Information

Galbanum oil is distilled from the milky oleoresin of members of the ferula plant species, including *Ferula galbaniflua*, which grow in the mountains of Northern Iran. Incisions are made near the base of the plant's stem to release the aromatic resin, which is then collected. *F. galbaniflua* can grow up to 2 metres (6 feet) tall and bears white umbelliferous flowers.

Galbanum's Legendary Power

Galbanum oil was celebrated in ancient times for its ritualistic and mystical qualities, because it has slightly narcotic properties that can induce a dreamy state. It was mentioned in the Bible as one of the sweet spices used to make holy incense. The ancient Egyptians and Romans used it as incense, too, also valuing it as an embalming agent, in addition to using it for cosmetic and perfumery purposes.

This is an extremely powerful oil for sacred work, yet very little has been written about this aspect of its nature. This is probably to prevent its power from falling into the wrong hands.

Some sources say that Morgan le Fey, a legendary British soul midwife associated with King Arthur and his lineage in the Isle of Avalon, used Galbanum as an anointing oil when she worked with the dying.

Galbanum's Esoteric Qualities

One of Galbanum's properties is that it allows us to expand our 'light body' in order to open portals. (Portals are two-way interdimensional doors opening into other realities.) Therefore, we should always use caution when working with this oil, because its energy field is so very powerful.

In addition to its work as a psychopomp, Galbanum is a great teacher of the soul and may reveal secrets to you. These could be anything from aspects of your own shadow to insights into past lives (which may trigger painful memories) or information from etheric time warps.

Galbanum is an oil for very experienced spiritual practitioners, so shouldn't be used lightly, frivolously or by anyone who's unused to this sort of work.

When to Use Galbanum

You can call on Galbanum for help when you need to initiate conversations with the dead, the newly dead and also ancestors. In addition, it will help the souls of those who have committed suicide to understand where they are in the afterlife. When appropriate, it can be used to perform healing rituals for them.

Galbanum can even be used to heal the soul trauma felt by someone who died unexpectedly. For instance, they may have left their earthly body very rapidly or shockingly as a result of an accident, if their death was very sudden or if they died at the hands of others. In addition, it's very soothing for anyone who died while experiencing immense fear or shock.

Karmic Roots

Galbanum has karmic links with Sirius.

Known as the Dog Star, Sirius is not only the brightest star in the constellation Canis Major, but also the brightest star in the night sky. Sirius was essential to ancient Egyptian mythology. One of the many theories about the Great Pyramid of Giza is that its southern shaft was constructed in perfect alignment with Sirius. The star was also associated with Isis, the Egyptian mother goddess. Many esoteric societies believe Sirius to be the home of the great metaphysical and spiritual teachers who have lived on Earth.

Guided Meditation

You might like to record this meditation before meditating with Galbanum. This will enable you to relax and listen to the meditation without unnecessary distractions. Simply follow the instructions for preparing yourself for a guided meditation (*see page 35*).

> *I'm the master of the threshold. With my guidance, it's possible to enter interdimensional doorways, so that we may communicate and interact with the spirits and souls of the dead.*
>
> *There may have been a gradual distancing from the Primordial Source for the soul you're guiding, where the veils between the realms of spirit and matter may have become sticky with tangled energy and now need to be cleared.*
>
> *We open the portals with pure, brilliant light, with interdimensional beings as our guides. Their level of spiritual evolution is beyond human understanding, but you may learn from them and speak the mutual language of the Divine to understand the plan of the cosmos.*
>
> *You'll receive all of the gifts you need both for this journey and for this divine work. And so may it be.*

Galbanum's Key Points

◊ Assists in soul ritual work

◊ Can form a bridge between the living and the dead

◊ For easing soul trauma for the dead

◊ Scent – fresh green top note with a woody undercurrent

◊ Affinity with the crown chakra

Contraindications

◊ Galbanum is an emmenagogue (able to help or induce menstruation), so should be avoided during pregnancy.

◊ This is a very sacred oil and should be treated with respect. It should only be used by very experienced practitioners.

CASE STUDY

Clive and Linda lived in a picture-postcard thatched cottage in Dorset, UK. Although their home was down a quiet country lane that was peaceful at night, they both suffered from vivid nightmares involving noisy battle scenes, horses and men being slain, fighting and bloodshed. Several times each week, they'd wake up clinging to each other in fear.

'What can be happening?' Linda asked when I bumped into her in our village shop. 'We've even stopped eating snacks in the evening in case it's a food intolerance.'

She invited me back for a coffee to see if I could sense anything unusual in the cottage. It all seemed peaceful and cosy, and her cats were friendly and content, asleep in the kitchen. (This is usually a good sign.)

I had a bottle of Galbanum with me. After we'd drunk our coffee, we sat quietly, placed a few drops of Galbanum on our foreheads (thereby activating the third eye) and tuned in to a deeper space.

Almost immediately, I heard a man shouting instructions. I felt stones and rocks flying over my head, and heard the thundering of horses' hooves nearby. There was a smell of blood and gunpowder, followed by a series of loud bangs. I withdrew from the scene as soon as I could, as did Linda.

Suddenly, it all made sense. A battle had been fought on Clive and Linda's land, and many souls were still stuck there, not realizing what had happened to them. I went back the following week, and used Galbanum in a releasing and blessing ritual to send the souls into the light.

Linda did some research at the County Records Office. She discovered that more than 100 men from our village had been injured or killed when protecting the local manor house from a *sudden attack during the English Civil War. As a result of our intervention, Clive and Linda are now sleeping much easier in their beds at night.*

. . . .

Holy Basil

Reconnecting with
the Divine Life Force

'Instead of worrying about what you cannot control,
shift your energy to what you can create.'
ROY T. BENNETT, *THE LIGHT IN THE HEART*

B asil has been cultivated for over 5,000 years, giving it an ancient and colourful healing lineage. Basil oil's high vibrational energy is uplifting, which makes it a powerful agent for enhancing the flow of the 'qi' life force. It stimulates creativity and increases concentration. It's also an oil that wakes up the soul and refreshes the spirit like a breath of fresh air.

Botanical Information

There are over 100 varieties of basil, each with a slightly different aroma. Every type of basil smells refreshing and they all share the same green, aromatic, spicy and herby scent that acts as a tonic for the soul and spirit. The plants are eaten as herbs, and their leaves add colour, flavour and a wide range of nutrients to foods. Yet, the herb known as Holy Basil (*Ocimum tenuiflorum*) has something extra – a focused and high vibration that kick-starts our sacred inner fire.

Holy Basil's Legendary Power

Holy Basil is beloved in several spiritual and religious traditions for its sacred connections, but especially in Hinduism, where it's still regarded as one of the most important plants in Ayurvedic medicine, renowned for healing both body and soul...

In India, Holy Basil is called *tulsi*, which is a Sanskrit word meaning 'incomparable one'. Many Hindu homes have *tulsi* plants growing close to the front door to attract high energy and prosperity into the household. Basil is also grown within the courtyards of temples. In the town of Varanasi, India, which is known for its care of the dead and dying, people very close to the end of life are splashed with water mixed with basil leaves to help to raise their departing souls to heaven.

Certainly, Holy Basil oil's high vibration aids the transition process on an energetic level by giving people the energy to die consciously, making it an important oil for soul midwives to use to help their patients.

Holy Basil's Esoteric Qualities

In esoteric terms, Holy Basil's energy is connected with inspiration, as well as the will to live and create with the divine force. The word 'inspire' comes from the Greek word *pneuma*, meaning 'to breathe'. When we're lacking in joy, feeling sullen and tired of the world, our breathing becomes shallow. Holy Basil creates the energy to breathe deeply, transforming our lethargy so we can recover our ecstatic inspiration.

The energies from Holy Basil affect us in several different ways, including opening the crown chakra and enhancing our power. This is useful for increasing feelings of self-worth when we've suffered abuse of any kind.

The oil can also be used to cut and clear energy in rituals that involve the releasing and cutting of ties that bind people together in a destructive relationship. In addition, it can be used to heal rifts and foster harmony between people who are ill at ease with each other.

For personal development work, Holy Basil can help us to open our third eye in order to gain inner vision, helping us to view situations and challenges from a different perspective.

When to Use Holy Basil

This oil is known to enhance personal power in order to bring self-awareness and clarity. It helps to dissolve negative relationships, first by encouraging us to realize that there's a problem, and secondly by giving us the courage and strength to separate from these difficult connections.

In esoteric work, such as conducting the souls of the dead (psychopomp work), it can act as a gatekeeper oil (*see page 31*), guarding the threshold between this world and the next.

Holy Basil oil can be used for protection before performing a ritual. It can also help to ease the passage in any situation where the soul is travelling during meditation or dreamwork.

Karmic Roots

Holy Basil oil has a very high vibration. It's multidimensional and opens portals into other realms, such as the devic realm. It has karmic connections with the planet Mercury and the god Hermes.

Mercury

This small planet, which is never more than 28 degrees from the Sun, is the messenger of the zodiac, just as the god for which it's named was the messenger of the gods. Mercury's close proximity to the Sun means that, at its highest level, it enables us to express our solar consciousness – our life's purpose. Mercury rules all forms of communication, whether they're physical or mental. Therefore, it controls our ability to think, talk to other people, process our ideas and assemble pieces of information into a coherent whole. Mercury is the ruling planet of Gemini (where he brings inquisitiveness, mental agility and chattiness) and Virgo (where he fosters a more practical and organized way of communicating).

Hermes

Mischievous Hermes was the messenger god of the Greeks and was known to the Romans as Mercury. He wore winged sandals, called talaria, which made him fleet of foot, and carried a staff or caduceus entwined with two serpents. Hermes guided travellers, whether they were gods or mortals, and was the guardian of transitions and crossroads. One of his most important roles was as a psychopomp or 'conductor of souls', as he escorted souls to Hades and sometimes, as in the case of Persephone, away from Hades and back to the world of the living.

Guided Meditation

To prepare yourself for a guided meditation, simply follow the instructions given (*see page 35*).

For a shorter meditation involving Holy Basil, you can place a few drops of the oil on your heart chakra, and meditate for five minutes at the beginning and end of each day, to receive energy and inspired thoughts.

Breathe in the colour green as you meditate with me, so you can see the portal into other dimensions of reality, glimpsing the great light beings who help us from the higher planes of consciousness.

When your world feels lacklustre, dull and stale, work with me to release old spiritual blockages and ancestral patterning that must be dissolved to make space for the new.

I'll help you to take responsibility for new and invigorating thoughts, feelings and actions. I can heal outdated karmic patterns that are hindering harmony within your relationships.

I'll scour away the residue from past lifetimes or your childhood and help you to reset your DNA, so you move towards becoming a fully conscious human being who's in alignment with your soul's purpose.

Work with me to learn how to take responsibility for your personal power and how it affects the life path of others.

I draw on energy from your etheric body to raise the frequency of your physical body, so as to restore compassionate love for your deep and immortal self.

Holy Basil's Key Points

◊ A gatekeeper oil

◊ Helps to dissolve difficult relationships

◊ Helps to cut emotional ties that are negative

124

◊ Scent – green, aromatic, spicy, reminiscent of cloves

◊ Affinity with the crown chakra

Contraindications

Holy Basil is an emmenagogue (it can induce or help menstruation), so shouldn't be used during pregnancy.

CASE STUDY

After five years of managing the creative team in an international advertising company, Steven was feeling dull and burned out. He didn't admit this to his colleagues, but his creative energy was at an all-time low and he felt he'd nothing left to offer. Despite this, he'd been offered a promotion and a large pay increase, so he could launch a new product. Although this gave Steven a much-needed confidence boost, and validated his expertise, he was anxious that the team would soon notice how tired he was on the inside.

Steven was struggling to keep up with the complexity of his workload three months into the job, which is when he made an appointment to see me on the recommendation of his yoga teacher.

'How can I get my spark back?' he asked me.

I suggested Holy Basil. Steven began by rubbing diluted Basil oil on the palms of his hands and breathing in the scent. He did this several times a day, with the intention of strengthening his aura. Holy Basil has a powerful link with the breath and is often used in conjunction with yoga.

The transformative green energy of Holy Basil invigorated Steven's chakras, opening his lungs wide, and he breathed in gulps of invigorating fresh air. His energy field strengthened as his vibration expanded, enabling him to think outside the box and visualize how to create change. He was soon bringing new and fresh ideas to his creative team.

Holy Basil dissolved the stagnant overwhelm in his head, enabling him to focus on bringing new zest and inspiration into his life.

He also rearranged the office and introduced Holy Basil oil in diffusers for a week; note of caution: it is best not to do this if you have pregnant women in the office, although the amounts of actual oil in the air would be extremely small. The effects of the oil became noticeable among his team, who also became more alert and curious, full of new and sparkling ideas. In essence, they all woke up to their potential which, like Steven's, had gone to sleep through repetition and stagnation.

The product launch was a great success and once more, Steven was riding high. 'The more breath I took, boosted by the sweet smell of Holy Basil, the more consciously I breathed the life force back into myself. I feel reborn!'

. . . .

Marigold

Vision and Prophecy

'Do not argue with what is, simply
follow the progress of truth.'
SUI/FOLLOWING, *I CHING*

Marigold positively shimmers with energy. It opens portals
to other worlds and often triggers a breakthrough
from one level of consciousness to another. It spans so many
dimensions that it's impossible to imagine its limits, because it's
both timeless and vast. Marigold is a wonderful oil for people
who have been working with such energy that they now feel
exhausted – it slowly brings them down from great heights. It
can also encourage dreams and daytime visions. Vibrant yellow
and gold in colour, it brings a sense of warmth and joy, as well as
a feminine energy that's nurturing and uplifting.

Botanical Information

This oil is distilled from the bright orange petals of *Calendula officinalis*, known as the pot marigold. It was called calendula, from the Latin *calendae*, which means the first day of the month, because it can flower from early June until November or even later in the northern hemisphere. *Officinalis* indicates that the plant was once sold by apothecaries because of its medicinal properties. The oil is sticky and viscous, and has a pungent musky scent.

When buying Marigold oil, it's essential to check which plant it's made from, as it can also be distilled from *Tagetes*, commonly known as African or French marigold. This is an entirely different species and its oil doesn't have the sacred properties of Calendula oil.

Marigold's Legendary Power

The marigold has long been regarded as a holy flower all over the world. Marigold flowers were sacred to the Aztecs, who believed that an essence made from them was a cure for being struck by lightning. The essence was also used in many religious ceremonies and rituals to evoke high energy.

In Mexico, marigold flowers are used during *Diá de los Muertos* – the Day of the Dead. This is celebrated on 1 November to honour all ancestors, especially any family and friends who have died in the last year. Marigolds are strewn on graves and on home altars to guide the dead souls back to their relatives. The dead souls are said to be attracted by the strong aroma of the flowers.

In Indian culture, it's believed that the liquid that results from steeping marigold petals in spring water can invoke psychic visions of fairies when rubbed on the eyes.

Marigold's Esoteric Qualities

This is one of several oils to have an etheric link to the temple teachings of Mary Magdalene, who's the mother of the myrrhophores. It represents her guidance and wisdom, and can be used to channel her teachings about working with all of the sacred oils. Marigold oil can act as a portal to her temple.

Marigold oil has been used for divination and healing for thousands of years. The wisdom it contains can form a mirror that reveals our true path and links us to parts of ourselves that may exist in a different dimension. (Some esoteric traditions maintain that we have an over-soul, which can exist simultaneously in other realms and lifetimes.) It's an all-seeing and all-knowing oil.

When to Use Marigold

This is an oil to use when you need to get to the root of something, because it gives insights in order to understand what you need to know. It can help in many difficult situations, including abuse (whether giving protection from abuse or balance after it), emotional trauma, fear, grief, sorrow, guilt, heartache and jealousy. Marigold can give protection from negative emotions, whether these are other people's or our own, and it's an excellent oil when we need to clear a situation or show forgiveness towards someone.

Marigold is invaluable for looking into the future for specific information about an event or when we want to know the outcome to a problem. The information will be given to us on a need-to-know basis, often in the form of images, which we then need to think about and meditate on in order to understand them better.

Karmic Roots

Marigold oil is connected with the Sun and Mary Magdalene.

The Sun

The Sun is the star at the centre of our solar system and is therefore essential to life. We rely on its warmth and light for our existence. In astrology, the Sun is the ruler of Leo and describes our life's purpose.

This oil has many links, both botanical and esoteric, with the Sun. Because calendula flowers are heliotropic (the flower heads move as they follow the course of the Sun throughout the day), they have a natural association with the Sun. Their petals are arranged in two sets of florets – disc florets and ray florets – which together look like the Sun's rays.

Mary Magdalene

The name 'marigold' is a derivation of 'Mary's gold' and the Mary to whom this refers is Mary Magdalene. For centuries, she's been a misunderstood and maligned figure in the story of Jesus's life. She was a teacher and belonged to the lineage of the Egyptian mystery teachings of Isis. Her teachings are largely to do with energy work and transition at a deep soul level. She was a highly trained temple priestess and belonged to a long lineage of light workers. Her etheric temple can be reached with the help of oils and meditations (*see page 38*).

Guided Meditation

You might like to record this meditation before meditating with Marigold. This will enable you to relax and listen to the meditation without unnecessary distractions. Simply follow the instructions for preparing yourself for a guided meditation (*see page 35*).

Use me to access the spiritual realms and to anchor yourself to star grids in other galaxies to bring in new information.

I bring strength, love and wisdom, so that you can work with new knowledge, absorbing and processing its meaning.

I'm an oil for healers and soul workers. I'll bring a shield of light to protect your aura and prevent your energy from being depleted or your soul space from being invaded when you're working deeply with the souls of others.

Work with me to magnify your energy field while you explore other dimensions in search of your soul essence.

I've been around for millions of years so, in my terms, the passing of decades is merely the blink of an eye. Working with me will offer you new ways of perceiving your life.

Gazing into the depths of my being offers you instant clarity and stillness of mind. By providing a point of soft focus, I'll help you to stay attentively in the present moment without judging it or needing it to change.

I'll help you to see with your third eye, so you can clearly perceive all that you need to see in order to spread your wings and grow.

Marigold's Key Points

◊ Enables us to get to the root of a problem or situation

◊ Protects against negative emotions

◊ Can give us insight into the future

◊ Scent – a very musky aroma

◊ Affinity with the brow chakra

Contraindications

◊ Oils from two different plants can be sold as 'Marigold', so check that the oil is made from *Calendula officinalis* before buying it.

◊ Marigold is an emmenagogue (it can induce or help menstruation), so shouldn't be used during pregnancy.

CASE STUDY

Seth was in a quandary. He'd recently met Kira, who was exactly 20 years younger than him, almost to the day. He couldn't put his finger on why she seemed so significant or why he felt they had an immediate recognition of each other on a soul level. It could have been to do with a past life, but he wasn't sure and confessed that he 'didn't trust' his feelings.

He hadn't even found Kira attractive when they first met. She was a bit too sweet and innocent for his taste, because he preferred women who were feisty and less deferential. Yet, there was something compelling and magnetic about her. Despite this, Seth felt strongly that he wasn't ready for commitment. Should he invest in their relationship or escape while he still could?

Seth needed to understand his connection to Kira, so he could have a spiritual rather than a physical perspective of a woman he'd never normally have been attracted to. For three days, he set aside time each morning to meditate and ask Marigold for guidance. He'd ask, 'Who is Kira? Why have we met? Why are we together now?' Marigold spoke to him each time, giving him all the answers he needed in a set of images that he then meditated on.

The first symbol he was given was a single soft pink rose, which made him realize that Kira was the essence of true love.

The second symbol took him into a room, where a curly-haired child lay on the floor, holding a book. The child looked just like Seth as a little boy. Was this his son?

The final image showed Seth's flat as being completely empty. No furniture, no books, no TV, no food in the fridge. It'd been emptied, as though someone else were about to move in. Instead of feeling upset, Seth sighed with relief. It was time to move on and he now knew who with.

Myrrh

Wisdom and Forgiveness

'And when they were come into the house, they saw the young child with Mary his mother, and fell down, and worshipped him: and when they had opened their treasures, they presented unto him gifts: gold and frankincense, and myrrh.'

MATTHEW 2:11

Myrrh is the guiding mother oil for myrrhophores or mistresses of the oils. Its spiritual qualities underpin the entire philosophy that oil priestesses aspire to: healing and serving humanity to raise consciousness.

Myrrh teaches us to practise wisdom and forgiveness, and to release negativity consciously in order to become a fully evolved master (or mistress). During temple training, a myrrhophore would be rigorously observed by her elders to check that she'd fully embraced this philosophy within her daily duties. This way, she could work with integrity to forgive those who'd sinned and to spread compassionate love into every aspect of their being.

The message that Myrrh sends us is that we may have all the material gifts in the world, but without love and forgiveness, we're nothing.

Botanical Information

Myrrh comes from the oleoresin produced by *Commiphora myrrha*, which is a small tree that grows up to 10 metres (33 feet) tall. It's native to Northeast Africa and Southwest Asia. Incisions are made into the bark of the tree with a specially designed knife to release the resin. This is exuded as a milky liquid that hardens into droplets or 'tears'. These are stored for about three months, during which time they dry out and their aroma gradually matures. The essential oil is created by steam distillation of this hardened resin.

Myrrh oil varies in colour from pale yellow to amber and has an earthy, slightly medicinal scent.

Myrrh's Legendary Power

Myrrh is an oil of great antiquity. It was used in incense and the earliest archaeological evidence of the incense trade is from South Arabia in about 6–5BCE.

It was also one of the main oils used for embalming by the ancient Egyptians. On the west bank of the Nile, at Thebes (known as the city of the dead), tombs were excavated, and traces of myrrh, juniper and cinnamon were discovered. During the embalming ceremony, the mortuary priests wore jackal heads in honour of the god Anubis. The priests would remove the brain and viscera from the corpse, chanting as they wrapped the body in linen bandages soaked in myrrh.

There's a legend that the Egyptian goddess Isis reassembled the dismembered body of her husband, Osiris, after it'd been cut to pieces by his brother, Set. Isis finally gave Osiris the gift of immortality by anointing his body with oils, chiefly Myrrh. He became the god of the underworld.

Myrrh also played an important role in Jesus's Nativity. The Magi, who followed the star to find the infant Jesus, are thought to have been Zoroastrian astrologer priests from Babylon, who understood the esoteric and healing properties of the gold, frankincense (*see page 101*) and myrrh that they took to the child.

This powerful oil was used in Europe as incense during funerals and cremations until the 15th century. It's the holy oil traditionally used in the Eastern Orthodox Church when administering the sacraments – commonly referred to as 'receiving the myrrh'. Accordingly, a mixture of wine and myrrh would have been offered to Jesus during the Crucifixion and was used by the myrrhophores (the three Marys) to anoint his dead body.

Myrrh's Esoteric Qualities

Myrrh brings wisdom and spiritual growth, as well as forgiveness. One of the first steps on the path to spiritual mastery and full empowerment is to learn how to connect to the Source of All in the correct manner. One element of this process is the soul's awakening. This prompts deep questions, such as, 'Who am I?', 'What am I here to do?' and 'How am I to serve?' Myrrh encourages this questioning process and, when used in meditation, gives us valuable insights.

Our spiritual gifts and abilities will become clear when we work with Myrrh and, once attuned to them, we'll become a channel to help lift the whole of humanity to higher levels of consciousness as we serve from the heart. This essentially means letting our heart guide our life, our thoughts and our actions.

Myrrh targets our fears and insecurities, challenging us to let them go and move on. If we can be strong and look into the heart of our darkness, we'll find nothing there to fear. Myrrh is the kindly teacher who releases us from our self-imposed prison into a new light, with room to grow.

When to Use Myrrh

Myrrh has a variety of important uses, all of which involve the process of release. It helps us to let go of our negative emotions, especially when we've been holding on to them for some time, when we're becoming aware of the harm they're causing both others and ourselves. Many of these emotions can stem from memories that are painful or that we've buried deeply within our psyches, so Myrrh gives us the courage to examine these difficult areas and begin to release them.

It also helps us to find it in our hearts to forgive anyone who's hurt or upset us, in addition to enabling us to forgive ourselves for our own actions and behaviour.

Karmic Roots

Myrrh has strong links with Frankincense (*see page 101*) and both oils are ruled by the planet Saturn (*see page 105*).

Guided Meditation

You might like to record this meditation before meditating with Myrrh. This will enable you to relax and listen to the meditation without unnecessary distractions. Simply follow the instructions for preparing yourself for a guided meditation (*see page 35*).

Never burden your heart with unreleased pain. It's toxic. Don't resist change. Instead, live with a calm and loving spirit. Ignore the demands of the ego and let go of all that no longer serves you.

Negative thoughts, fear of the future and mistrust of other people and difficult situations breed misunderstanding, anger and sadness. Let go and love instead.

Your own progress will be blocked if you cannot let go of dark thoughts, blame and anger. Meet everything with compassion and love. Become the sage that you are and the divine being that you truly are.

See and feel the pain you've caused through your own fear and confusion. Feel your own sorrow and regret. Sense that, finally, you can release this burden and ask for forgiveness, saying simply, 'I forgive myself.'

Think of your own precious life. Feel the sorrow you've carried from the past and know that you can release this burden of pain by extending forgiveness when your heart's ready.

Let yourself remember and visualize the ways that you've hurt others. Ask quietly for their forgiveness. As you understand the power of these actions, your wisdom will grow and your life will be changed forever.

Myrrh's Key Points

◊ Releases negative emotions

◊ Enables forgiveness of others and oneself

◊ One of the gifts from the Magi at the Nativity

◊ Scent – earthy, medicinal

◊ Colour – amber

◊ Affinity with the base, heart and throat chakras

Contraindications

◊ Myrrh is an emmenagogue (it can induce or help menstruation), so shouldn't be used during pregnancy.

◊ Myrrh shouldn't be used in conjunction with anticoagulants as it might interfere with medication.

CASE STUDY

Sometimes readers write to me. One email came from a man called Gus:

'I have an emotional problem that's really interfering with my life and it seems to be getting worse. I'm spiritual in my outlook and wonder if I should take my problems to a spiritual teacher of some kind or try to work through them on my own. I'm a very intense and extreme person. I'm also very impatient to work through this block. Would the sacred oils give me any answers?'

I felt that they could. At least Gus had realized that he did indeed have a problem and had begun to try to look for a solution. As he didn't give any other information about his problem, I dowsed for an oil that might help him and the pendulum hovered over Myrrh.

I noticed that Gus described himself as extreme and impatient. Extremes of any kind can create an imbalance that can upset a person's emotional, mental and physical health. The body has many natural mechanisms for bringing itself back into harmony. Extremes also cause blockages of energy that can manifest emotionally. In addition, I sensed that Gus was a perfectionist who lived off his nerves.

When I emailed Gus, I suggested that he work with Myrrh in meditation. I also recommended adding a few drops to his bathwater at night (having mixed it first with some milk to help it to dissolve in the water). This would help to wash away his worries. After a few weeks, he emailed with a progress report:

'I realized that I've been so "in my head" that I haven't been properly in my body for a long time. I think this stems from my mother dying two years ago. I've been so intent on working on this problem that I've set aside at least an hour a day for focused practice, as well as the baths.

'Almost immediately, I began to change my ideas about what I thought was causing the problem. I thought it was to do with grief, but then this subtly shifted and I realized it was tied up with a lot of anger that I'd kept inside and not fully expressed.

'I was raging that my mother had died and not said goodbye to me. One day she was there and full of life, and the next day she wasn't. (She died unexpectedly in her sleep.) We'd had no closure on certain longstanding difficulties between us and now there was *no chance to put that right. It was as if she'd left halfway through an important conversation.*

'As soon as I realized this, I knew I'd hit on the truth of why I was in such a state. I felt angry and abandoned. I know this sounds irrational, but why had she left in this way? I persevered with these insights. Over time, I realized that I needed not only to forgive her for going, but also to forgive myself. In truth, I knew that I hadn't given her as much time as she'd needed in her last months. I'd been so busy and had ignored her needs. She was desperate to see more of me and I just found other things to do.

'As you can see, I've been feeling a lot of guilt. The Myrrh somehow gave me the idea of creating a small ritual in which I lit a candle and talked to my mother as if she were in the room with me. I told her everything I was feeling and asked for her forgiveness. She was definitely there in spirit with me, listening to what I was saying. In return, she seemed to give me her forgiveness. I told her how much I loved and missed her (something I'd never quite managed to do while she was alive), and the energy in the room became soft and beautiful. I knew then that I could put this behind me and move on with my life. I've got Mum's photograph in my wallet. We've healed the rift and she's now with me all the time... and I've realized she didn't need to say goodbye because, actually, she never really left.'

. . . .

Myrtle

Gatekeeper of
the Sacred Threshold and
for Summoning the Muse

*'And they answered the angel of the Lord
that stood among the myrtle trees.'*
ZECHARIAH 1:11

Myrtle plays a very special role in helping us to access other realms and realities. We may wish to do this for our own spiritual growth, such as in shamanic work, in spirit rescue or if we're involved in psychopomp work. Before we do anything that involves spiritual travel into other dimensions, we need to contact the gatekeeper (*see page 31*) who guards the space that we want to access. As an ancient gatekeeper oil, Myrtle helps us to see the truth in all things and to make discerning choices in our spiritual quests.

Botanical Information

Myrtle oil is extracted by steam distillation from the fresh leaves of *Myrtus communis*, which is an aromatic shrub that grows up to 4 metres (13 feet) tall. It has small, shiny, fragrant dark green leaves and scented white flowers, bearing small black berries. *Myrtus communis* is native to Africa, but is now grown widely across both the Mediterranean and Europe.

The oil can be pale yellow or orange, and has a spicy and aromatic scent. It's mainly produced in Spain, Tunisia, Corsica, Italy and France.

Myrtle's Legendary Power

In ancient Egypt, myrtle was associated with the otherworld, serving as a reminder of the eternal life of the soul.

Myrtle has long been used for its healing properties, which include treating skin complaints and breathing problems. The ancient Egyptians treated infections and fevers with wine in which myrtle leaves had been steeped.

The plant is associated with the naked Aphrodite, who hid behind a myrtle bush on the island of Cythera, Greece, to cover her modesty. She was so grateful to the plant that she bestowed patronage on it, and it's always linked with her power of beauty and love. Myrtle was therefore used in ancient Greece in the rites of Aphrodite.

Myrtle is linked with bouquets carried by brides in the British royal family. In the language of flowers, myrtle represents love, so a few sprigs of the plant are often used in wedding bouquets. Sprigs cut from the myrtle bush growing in the gardens of Osborne House, Queen Victoria's home on the Isle of Wight, have featured in the bouquets of brides of the British royal family since 1858.

Myrtle's beneficial effects on the skin mean that its leaves and flowers were the main ingredients in *l'eau des anges*, or angels' water, which was manufactured in France in the 19th century as a cosmetic. In parts of France, myrtle is still planted as a herbal talisman to protect houses from the evil eye, but it's only thought to hold this protective power if it's planted by a woman.

Myrtle's Esoteric Qualities

Myrtle is a gatekeeper oil (*see page 31*), which means it can be used to guard thresholds. Its high vibration is transcendental and may be used to commune with the souls of the dead. It can also be used to explore previous incarnations through meditation or to give past-life readings. Myrtle is excellent for dreamwork, divination and prophecy.

Its energy vibrates at a very high frequency, and is delicate, devotional and very feminine. Myrtle enhances our intuition, creativity and, in some cases, clairvoyance. It's also a powerful oracle oil that can sharpen our vision when looking into the past or the future; this is because it straddles time.

This oil is a marvellous soul healer. It may also be very helpful in cases of trauma, fear, self-destructive tendencies and feelings of hopelessness.

When to Use Myrtle

The power of Myrtle should never be underestimated. It's invaluable when you're doing deep work, not only because of its ability to make contact with other realms and connections to discarnate beings, but also because of its role as a guardian or gatekeeper.

Myrtle brings insight into, and greater understanding of, knowledge, thereby enriching and deepening our grasp of important or complex topics.

This is a very feminine oil, so is excellent at fostering intuition and love. It soothes troubled emotions and helps in the search for truth. Myrtle promotes self-love and self-acceptance, so can support anyone who's feeling an element of self-hatred or self-disgust.

Karmic Roots

Myrtle is connected to the planets Venus and Neptune.

Venus

The planet Venus is named after the Roman goddess Venus, who was Aphrodite in Greek mythology. In astrology, Venus is known as the planet of love and beauty. Venus encourages us to create loving bonds with other people. It's one of the personal planets, which means that its position in our birth chart has a major influence on our character. Venus is the ruling planet of Taurus (where she exerts a tactile and sensuous influence) and Libra (where she strives for harmony and diplomacy).

Neptune

Neptune is the planet of mystery and is known as the higher octave of Venus. Astrologically, Neptune has no boundaries, so it rules the numinous and the invisible, fostering a great understanding of the unseen or sowing seeds of confusion and doubt. It's named after the god of the sea, known as Neptune to the Romans and Poseidon to the Greeks.

Neptune is one of the three outer planets. Because it moves so slowly through the solar system, completing its orbit of the Sun once every 165 years, it has a generational influence on us. It's the ruling planet of Pisces, which is the sign of the Fish and therefore very attuned to Neptune's watery depths.

Myrtle's Key Points

◊ The prime gatekeeper oil

◊ Enhances intuition

◊ Can boost psychic abilities

◊ Encourages stable emotions

◊ Scent – spicy and aromatic

◊ Affinity with the brow chakra

Contraindications

Myrtle is an emmenagogue (it can induce or help menstruation), so shouldn't be used during pregnancy.

Guided Meditation

You might like to record this meditation before meditating with Myrtle. This will enable you to relax and listen to the meditation without unnecessary distractions. Simply follow the instructions for preparing yourself for a guided meditation (*see page 35*).

> *I, the spirit of Myrtle, have worked with visionary activity for thousands of years. I help to strengthen the aura, gently opening the third eye in order to see things in a new way. As you become*

more aware of these subtle energies surrounding you, you'll be filled with light.

I can transfer consciousness from the Divine into your own consciousness as you awaken spiritually. As you dream at night, I'll be working with you to bring you new information and understanding.

I may enable you to receive psychic abilities, such as telepathy, psychometry and remote viewing to bring another perspective to your understanding. I can unblock old subconscious patterns and bring emotional stability while you make leaps in understanding of complex matters. We all need to see the truth in all things, because it gives us power and discernment.

CASE STUDY

Calling in the muse is a process that's familiar to all creative people. Penelope, a writer in her thirties, was about to start writing a new book – a fantasy novel based on Greek myths.

She'd spent months devising the story and crafting characters, and was always beavering away. But something was missing. The plot, which had seemed so exciting in her imagination, was looking dry and staid, and no 'magic' was springing from the page. She explained it to me thus: 'If it looks lacklustre to me, what on earth will the readers think of it?'

Then, during some research into the early Olympians, Penelope saw a reference to myrtle sprigs being used in the wreaths of emperors, suggesting that the scent was used to give them creativity and inspiration. With nothing to lose, Penelope ordered a bottle of Myrtle oil and meditated with it twice a day.

An astonishing thing happened. Her hero, who was the leading character in her book, tapped her arm while she was asleep in bed and started talking to her.

'At first I thought it was a lucid dream, but he was so real that I could feel his breath and see the colour of his eyes. He described scenes and events from the book, suggesting some changes to spice things up a bit. He also told me a little about his family, things that I could never have imagined and that brought a completely new slant to the story. It was totally bizarre. I've heard of characters coming to life, but didn't believe it could really happen. His suggestions added so much colour, vitality and vivacity to the novel that I ended up rewriting every word.

'He told me that Myrtle had summoned him to be of service to me while I meditated. Had I channelled a spirit who had a story to tell? Or had I created a persona that came to life? I'll never know.'

. . . .

Opoponax

Shape-shifting and Shape-borrowing

'Granny Weatherwax had many times flicked
through the channels of consciousness around her...
to listen with the body of a beetle, so that the world
is a three-dimensional pattern of vibrations.'
TERRY PRATCHETT, *LORDS AND LADIES*

Opoponax is a magical oil that's always been associated with wise women, and the arts of shape-shifting and shape-borrowing. Shape-shifting, which involves taking on the forms of other beings such as animals, birds and even plants, gives us insights into that of the animals', birds' and plants' unique ways and wisdom. It allows us to know what it's like to be in someone else's shoes and to learn the truth of true being. It's part of the journey of mastery.

This oil takes us on a magical journey during which we have to learn purity of heart and soul, compassion, love, wisdom and integrity. It's associated with the hero's quest and teaches us to check our path wisely. Above all, it teaches us to follow the path of the heart.

Botanical Information

Also known as sweet myrrh and bisabol myrrh, Opoponax oil is distilled from the oleoresin exuded from incisions made in the bark of trees from the *Commiphora* species, including *C. erythraea*. These trees are native to Somalia and eastern Ethiopia. They belong to the same family as *Commiphora myrrha*, from which Myrrh (*see page 135*) is extracted.

Opoponax's Legendary Power

King Solomon regarded Opoponax as one of the 'noblest' of all the incense gums. Various cultures used it to guard against negative influences, strengthen the senses, and increase awareness and intuition. This is an extremely powerful oil. If it calls you to work with it, you can be certain that your work will be of a very deep nature.

Opoponax's Esoteric Qualities

This oil calls you into sacred service. It creates a quickening in the spirit and a rush to begin our heroic mission – to leap across boundaries and feel no fear. It can whisper subtly or create a lion's roar so loud that we can't escape its message.

It takes tenacity and determination to link in with Opoponax, but it's a powerful oil that will teach us about transforming and transmuting power in order to discover our full destiny.

Opoponax connects with magical vision, in addition to the deep and sometimes dark feminine aspect of our lives. It can also attract luminous entities from all directions and other realms who come forward to share our journey. It has a strong affinity with snake medicine (transformational energy), which can push us out of our comfort zones, forcing us to show stealth and courage. It's an oil that we must respect, too. Work wisely with Opoponax and ask your gatekeeper to be vigilant in shielding you from the energies that you may encounter when opening your energetic field to this oil.

This oil helps you to navigate between the different worlds and outside time, showing you that there's a larger purpose in life, while revealing the grand and Divine plan for humanity. You need to tune in to this oil by discovering its sigils and sounds carefully and slowly over time (*see page 43*), and there's no quick route.

Opoponax has a theme, which is that as humans we've come out of alignment with the sacred. In addition, the balance between light and dark, masculine and feminine, is precarious. The outcome of this power struggle is by no means certain, although Opoponax is devoted to rebalancing and harmonizing the human psyche.

When to Use Opoponax

This oil gives us clarity. It exposes illusions, lies and false glamour, putting us on the path to truth. When we encounter obstacles along this path, Opoponax enables us to shape-shift our way through them. It cleanses our auric field. It also realigns us to spirit, enhances our spirituality and awareness, and gives us protection against negative energies.

When we need to lay down plans and cement them swiftly, Opoponax gives us the mental and physical energy that we need. When we need to shed old patterns, perhaps because they're holding us back, Opoponax can help.

Opoponax connects us to archetypes, including families of gods, angels and other light beings. It can also be used as an aid to divination and prophecy.

Karmic Roots

Opoponax has karmic links with the Moon and Hecate.

The Moon is the Earth's only natural satellite and we only ever see one of its faces. The other is always turned away from us, invisible in the dark.

Being such a visible part of our skies, the Moon has influenced many aspects of our lives for millennia, including the calendar (we divided the year up into months, based on the Moon's phases). It also regulates many biological cycles in the animal and plant kingdoms, and is known to affect the sleep patterns of many.

In astrology, the Moon governs our habits, instincts and needs, as well as our relationship with our mother. It's the ruler of Cancer, the sign of the crab - a reminder that the Moon influences the sea's tides.

Many of the world's cultures feature lunar goddesses. For the Greeks, there were three:

◊ Artemis, the maiden, who was linked with the Waxing Moon.

◊ Demeter, the mother, who was linked with the Full Moon.

◊ Hecate, the wise woman, who was linked with the Waning Moon.

The goddess Hecate is often depicted as having three heads, which enabled her to see in every direction at once. She was the goddess of the crossroads and although food was left for her in the past, present and future in order to honour her, her reach extended further than physical meeting points into the spiritual places of transition, including the sacred threshold between life and death.

Guided Meditation

You might like to record this meditation before meditating with Opoponax. This will enable you to relax and listen to the meditation without unnecessary distractions. Simply follow the instructions for preparing yourself for a guided meditation (*see page 35*).

I symbolize vision, death and the shadow. I can take you to the deepest mysteries in life, but you need to be ready to shed your own skin and release all that no longer serves you.

The spiral path of transformation, wisdom, understanding and wholeness is the magic cord by which the shaman travels to the soul world.

I'm the energy of wholeness and balance within cosmic consciousness, as well as the ability to experience anything willingly and without resistance. I'm the knowledge that all things are equal in creation, that all is one.

Use me to shed your illusions and limitations, so you can use your vitality and desires to achieve wholeness. When I come into your life, you can expect many changes. Forces may awaken. Your intuition will strengthen and sharpen.

Opoponax's Key Points

◊   Re-establishes balance and harmony

◊   Promotes clarity of thought

◊   Can attract luminous entities

◊   Encourages us to follow our hearts

◊   Scent – spicy, sweet and slightly floral, with woody, earthy notes

◊   Affinity with the base chakra

Contraindications

Opoponax is phototoxic (it reacts to ultraviolet light, causing possible blistering and inflammation of the skin), so shouldn't be applied directly to the skin.

CASE STUDY

Freya was a dedicated student of sacred oils, but had reached a plateau in her studies and felt blocked. Her understanding simply wasn't developing and she was only able to connect with the teachings about the oils in what felt like a superficial way.

A scientist by training, she admitted to being over-analytical at times and wasn't easily able to slip into heart space, which is so important when working with the oils.

'Intuition is something that doesn't seem to come naturally to me and "feeling" the energy of the oils is sometimes a challenge,' she explained. 'How can I learn to "feel" energy?'

Many students ask this question. Other than telling them to tune in, open up and receive the wisdom, there's no easy answer. In Freya's case, I suggested that she work with Opoponax, because it has such an affinity with snake medicine. Snakes are our best teachers for understanding vibration and energy. They don't have ears, and for their survival, they rely entirely on picking up the vibrations around them. Snakes are traditional 'familiars' of priestesses, who often wore their pet snake wrapped around their arms. They used snakes to give euthanasia to the dying, harvesting their venom that could be used to induce trances for channelling and prophecy. By shape-shifting into the world of the snake during meditation, we can begin to heighten our own sensitivity and resonance with vibration.

With some guidance, using a special mandala as a key to open the door, Freya worked with Opoponax and found herself slipping into snake spirit. Before long, she felt her energy field change, becoming fluid and slithery, like a snake rippling across the sand. Gradually, she began to sense the very subtle messages coming from the oils.

She explained, 'My sensitivity heightened and I could feel new ideas taking root within my body, which seemed to be the filter, rather than my mind, which had stopped asking so many insistent *questions. I also got a sense of how snakes shed their skins to cast off their past and change the future. It's given me a new understanding and an insight about the limitations that my mind had placed on me. I can now become a snake whenever I want to access an oil's wisdom and I'm no longer feeling blocked.'*

. . . .

Palo Santo

Protection

'May he grant that I see the sun-disc and behold the moon
unceasingly every day; may my soul go forth to travel to
every place which it desires; may my name be called out,
may it be found at the board of offerings; may there be given
to me loaves in the Presence like the Followers of Horus.'

SPELL 15, PAPYRUS OF ANI, FROM *THE ANCIENT EGYPTIAN
BOOK OF THE DEAD*, TRANSLATED BY R.O. FAULKNER

Palo Santo, whose name means 'holy wood', is an extremely powerful oil for psychic protection and is therefore essential for anyone involved in any type of soul work. This includes healing, working as a psychopomp, shamanic work and any other activity that brings us in contact with the deepest depths of the psyche, whether it's other people's or our own.

This pungent-selling oil serves to protect us from negative energy that might surround us in buildings and crowded spaces, especially hospitals, hospices and prisons. It's also useful for providing protection on public transport, where there's usually a mixture of intense energies. In addition, Palo Santo can help us when dealing with negative people and toxic relationships.

Botanical Information

In keeping with its mysterious character, palo santo has a very interesting botanical background. The palo santo tree (*Bursera graveolens*) grows widely across South America, but is commercially harvested chiefly in Ecuador. The essential oil is distilled from the heartwood of dead and fallen branches of the palo santo tree. After the wood has fallen it continues to mature, enabling the oil to develop in the heartwood as the timber dries out. The oil becomes more powerful the longer the wood is left – higher-quality oil comes from heartwood that's at least two years old.

Ecuadorian plant shamans say that the spirits of the sacred palo santo trees transmute the energy of the dead wood into the healing oil, which gives it its powerful protective properties.

Palo Santo's Legendary Power

This oil has been in indigenous South American shamanic use since time immemorial. Earliest written documents reveal that the Incas used it as a protective, purifying and ritualistic oil when establishing the Incan Empire in what is now Peru, between AD1438–1533.

The Incas revered many gods, including Inti, the Sun god, who was usually depicted in human form, his face a golden disc from which rays and flames flared out. Although he could be generous and benevolent, he was also feared. This was because the Incas believed that solar eclipses were the manifestation of his anger. They would give him offerings of palo santo to appease this destructive aspect.

Palo Santo's Esoteric Qualities

Palo Santo is still widely used within shamanic practice. In Ecuador and Peru, it's revered for banishing *mala energía* (bad energy), in addition to coaxing away demons and other negative influences, from both people and buildings.

Palo santo wood is often burned as incense and used to smudge a person's energy field to release the evil spirits attached to them that may be causing an illness. Myrrhophores use the oil, diluted in rapeseed oil and stroked through the aura, to cleanse a patient and remove any spirit attachments.

Associated as it is with the Sun, Palo Santo represents dragon energy, which holds the combination of dark and light, male and female, yin and yang. The dragon's fiery zest repels negativity and anchors the light, so that healing can take place.

In ancient wisdom, fire represents the boundary between the physical and etheric planes. Initiates accessed the spiritual realm through fire (hence a baptism of fire), such as fire-walking or sitting around a fire. Even lighting a candle creates the connection with fire, which is why candles are lit in churches to aid contemplation and prayer, and to call in the Divine. Working with Palo Santo in meditation, for personal growth, may also give us the sense that we've entered another dimension of reality.

When to Use Palo Santo

Palo Santo is one of the most powerful oils that I work with. I call it spiritual disinfectant. You can sweep it through your aura whenever you're exposed to negative energy. It's invaluable for healers and soul workers. This is because it creates a shield of light throughout the aura to prevent the depletion or invasion of their personal space. It's a wonderful healer of psychic wounds, repairing holes in the aura that may have been caused by trauma or soul loss.

During periods of intense spiritual enquiry or exploration, Palo Santo anchors our feet firmly on the ground, keeping us in line with our soul's purpose. It can also be used to lift curses, and to enhance prayer, ritual and other energy work.

Karmic Roots

Palo Santo has karmic links with the Sun.

The spurts of energy, known as spicules and prominences, erupting inside the Sun's corona look like flames to us on Earth, extending thousands of kilometres into space. Solar flares, which shoot atomic particles into space at vast speeds, can affect both weather systems and power grids on Earth. In astrology, the Sun is the ruler of Leo and describes our life's purpose.

Guided Meditation

You might like to record this meditation before meditating with Palo Santo. This will enable you to relax and listen to the meditation without unnecessary distractions. Simply follow the instructions for preparing yourself for a guided meditation (*see page 35*).

I'm Palo Santo, the strong dark force for good, offering strength and protection from darkness. I'm here to shine a light in dark places. Wherever you use me, I bring strength and love and deep protection. I'm a mighty warrior, my essence bringing thunder and lightning to your energy field, casting out demons.

Call on me when you need a barrier to protect you against another's energy. If you're working with the sick, I'll stop their illness from being absorbed by you.

I'll hold your hand in busy, anxious places where there are many people. I'll be with you as you offer deep work, holding the soul of another. I'll transmute darkness, sadness and soul pain. And I'll be the loving and strong pair of hands that will keep you safe from all that's not helpful or of the light.

Palo Santo's Key Points

◊ For deep soul work (whether for others or yourself)

◊ For psychopomp work

◊ For working with people at the end of life

◊ For dealing with people suffering from psychic attack

◊ For clearing your home's energies

◊ For clearing the space before a ritual

◊ For clearing toxic energy and as a barrier when coping with toxic relationships

◊ Scent – pungent

◊ Affinity with the base chakra

Contraindications

◊ Should only be bought from reputable sources that protect the environment in which it grows. The oil is harvested from the heartwood of the dead tree and is expensive to buy. Be wary of adulterated versions.

◊ May cause sensitivities in some people.

CASE STUDY

*Many healers are empaths, soaking up the pain and emotions
of the people they're trying to help. Without even noticing, they
absorb the energy around them.*

*Sarah was a psychiatric nurse working in an acute psychiatric
unit. She asked for help after coping with chronic exhaustion and
a series of viral illnesses and infections. After developing her latest
illness, she explained to me that she wasn't able to 'shake this
thing off'. Listening to her words and noticing her heavy shoulders
and the weariness in her voice, I could see that she was indeed
burdened by heavy and sticky negative energy.*

*Given the nature of Sarah's work, it was easy to see that she might
have absorbed a lot of the trauma experienced by her patients, who
were often in extreme chaos and disturbance. Sarah admitted that
she didn't do any energy clearing for herself because she was always
too tired to remember.*

*Because of this, we began with a healing session. I drew in the
light and asked Sarah's own guides to help her to release the energy
in her field that wasn't serving her highest good. We then called in
the spirit of Palo Santo to assist in dispelling, with love, any last
deep traces of spirit that might be clinging on to Sarah's subtle
bodies. Using Palo Santo on my hands, I worked throughout her
energy field, drawing the energy from her, using my thumbs and*

index fingers in a spinning motion, working through her chakras to replace the dark energy with blasts of pure white light.

We did this once a week for over a month. Each day before Sarah went to work, she'd also use Palo Santo to cleanse and protect herself. This would be repeated before bedtime.

Sarah began to notice a difference almost immediately. The first change was that her sense of humour returned and she'd started laughing again. She hadn't realized how heavy her moods had become. As Sarah continued to recover her life force she realized how much she still needed protection, not only from her patients, but also from many other situations around her that were draining her of energy – and she was able to find this with Palo Santo.

. . . .

Patchouli

Grounding

'The shock of unsettling events brings fear and trembling.
Move towards a higher truth and all will be well.'
CHÊN/THE AROUSING, *I CHING*

Patchouli has a solid and low vibration, which makes it a steady and useful member of the sacred oils repertoire. It's a wonderful oil for bringing us back to earth if we've been working with other oils of a very high vibration, because these can make us feel 'out of body' and unearthed.

Working with Patchouli is like taking a deep breath and putting on a pair of lead boots, especially after doing a lot of esoteric work. It pulls us back down to earth, slows our vibration and restores our links with the ordinary world. I'm sure this is why it was loved and used so much by hippies and the flower power movement in the 1960s, when recreational drugs were being experimented with, leaving many people with psychic burn-out and an overload from the energy of psychotropic drugs such as LSD. Patchouli, with its deep grounding properties, puts us right back in our body, calming and restoring our aura.

Botanical Information

The patchouli shrub (*Pogostemon cablin*) is native to Malaysia, but is cultivated for its oil in other parts of Asia as well, including Indonesia and China. It grows up to 3 metres (10 feet) tall, bearing white flowers with a purple tinge, and has large, fragrant leaves that release their warm, rich and spicy scent when rubbed. The essential oil is steam distilled from the leaves and shoots, and is either yellowy-brown or greeny-brown in colour.

Patchouli's Legendary Power

Patchouli is so connected with the Earth and feminine energy that its history and mythology are closely woven in with the archetype of Gaia, who was the mother of all of the Greek gods.

Legend states that Tutankhamun, the boy king of ancient Egypt, was buried with jars containing several gallons of Patchouli oil. Patchouli is associated with money and abundance in Indian legends. This was underlined in the 18th and 19th centuries, when dried patchouli leaves were tucked into the folds of Indian silks and other expensive fabrics before they were exported to wealthy purchasers in the West, believed to protect the fabrics against damage from moths and other insects.

Patchouli's Esoteric Qualities

Its grounding qualities make Patchouli oil one of the masters of transmutation. It can help us to work with high energies from other dimensions and bring them down to a safer level. Patchouli stops us from blowing a psychic gasket.

Despite its grounding qualities, Patchouli also stimulates super-consciousness without it overloading our system. In this way, it enables future collective consciousness to be understood and processed (during meditation or astral travel), and then stored in cellular data banks within the body for retrieval later.

At a simpler level, Patchouli oil increases the ability to recall past incarnations, particularly those involving the Himalayas. Sometimes these past lives may even involve being a different life form, such as an extraterrestrial.

Working with Patchouli as a master teacher can enhance our ability to see the bigger picture of life. It allows us to make a rapid alignment with our soul's purpose by both calling in and manifesting the things we need to see and work on.

In a base way, this could involve attracting the material things that we want (or think we want) in life. But in its highest and most sacred use, it often works by encouraging us to enter a temporary period of sacrifice or difficulty in order to achieve and fully integrate our supreme soul mission.

Patchouli releases emotional confusion and stops jitteriness after heightened experiences such as telepathy, psychic work and levitation. It will gradually calm the aura when it's been extended too widely and too quickly.

When to Use Patchouli

Whenever we've overstretched ourselves and feel fragile, wobbly and vulnerable, or when we're out of balance and out of our natural rhythm, Patchouli will put us back on our feet again. It's also an oil to use when suffering from mental exhaustion.

Patchouli helps to combat narcissistic behaviour, whether it is someone else's or our own. In addition, it balances mood swings.

If we've left our body as a result of drugs or extreme psychic activities, Patchouli will gently but firmly bring us back into our body again. It can be used when working with disruptive spirits and entities, not only for protection, but also to keep us steady and focused. When we've been working with high levels of energy, Patchouli anchors us back to the earth, because it nurtures and grounds us. It can be used to enhance our spiritual growth.

Karmic Roots

Patchouli's karmic roots lie with the Earth (*see page 78*) and with Gaia.

Greek mythology tells us that Gaia, or Mother Earth, was born after the vast space of Chaos was created. She was the first of the gods, giving birth to the sky, the mountains and the sea. Everything that followed did so because of her original creations. She was literally the earth mother.

Inspired by this myth, the chemist James Lovelock developed the Gaia hypothesis in the 1970s. This proposed that the Earth has a global consciousness and that life is a self-regulating system in which all living things interact with their environment to maintain perfect conditions for life on our planet. Without this global consciousness, we're lost.

Guided Meditation

You might like to record this meditation before meditating with Patchouli oil. This will enable you to relax and listen to the meditation without unnecessary distractions. Simply follow the instructions for preparing yourself for a guided meditation (*see page 35*).

> *Go quietly, open your mind and see what's happening. Accept that there are lessons to learn and realize that you may be blocking*

energy rather than allowing it to flow with ease. Don't be tempted to slip into anger or blame, but see the blue sky beyond the storm, without exhausting yourself in your search. All will come to you in the fullness of time.

Purify your thoughts and actions, and deepen your roots into the earth in order to be nourished and made strong.

Sometimes we have to limit ourselves and reduce our power in order to heal. If you take a rest and then ask for what you need to enhance your journey again, I'll be here to help you to grow stronger and wiser, showing you opportunities that you never dreamed possible.

Patchouli's Key Points

◊   Grounding and stabilizing, especially after esoteric work

◊   Helps when recalling past lives

◊   Assists when working with high energies

◊   Helps to see the bigger picture

◊   Releases emotional confusion

◊   Combines well with Elemi (*see page 83*)

◊   Scent – warm, rich and spicy

◊   Affinity with the base chakra

Contraindications

It may very occasionally cause some sensitivity in some people, so should be used with caution at first.

CASE STUDY

Skakira is a priestess/shaman living on a remote Scottish island, where her work involves connecting people with their ancestors. She undertakes shamanic journeys for people, bringing back messages from their female family lines to help their inner growth. When I first saw her, Skakira had journeyed so far, and across so many thousands of years while she reconnected with spirit, that coming 'home' to this world was often a trial, leaving her feeling depleted and very alone.

She also had a sense of not wanting to return from her journeying fully. Shaman have a foot in both worlds and the lure of the otherworld can be very powerful, unless the re-entry to this reality is completely grounded. I felt that Patchouli oil, with its sacred gift of return and grounding after extreme psychic work, might be of help to her.

This is how Skakira described her experience of connecting with one of her own ancestral guides, which in turn linked her to the spirit of the oil:

'I met an old man. He was thin and gaunt and clothed in filthy rags. He had bones dangling from his tattered sleeves. His face changed with each visiting spirit. He was a wise ancestor, holding the stories of all of my forefathers, and he was the head of my tribe. In his pouch were pots of herbs, twigs and lichens. He was dark and shadowy, sitting in a circle of ash, which seemed to draw a protective ring around him.

'He spoke of spiritual challenges and as he did so, I felt an expanded wisdom and deeper understanding of what had been happening to me and my own soul while travelling for others. I realized that I'd left aspects of my soul in the ancestral world and needed to reclaim them as soon as I could. A shamanic friend worked with me to retrieve this lost "essence" of myself and the spirit of Patchouli guarded the space for us while the return took place.

'Now, Patchouli calls me home when I've journeyed too far and for too long. It not only brought me the power to seek change, but also the knowledge that the seeker never stands alone, because our guides are there when we call for them. Patchouli oil is now my protective talisman.'

. . . .

Ravensara

Healing Soul Wounds

'Father, my heart is broken. I feel like it is in pieces.
I need to put my heart into your care. Will you
take care of it for me? I want to be able to love
again. I don't want to be bitter and brittle.'

ANONYMOUS,
PRAYER FOR HEALING A BROKEN HEART

When the soul is wounded in some way, the pain affects every aspect of our lives, whether we're conscious of it or not. Soul wounds are part of the human condition and I like to think of them as pain that happens for a reason. They help to ripen our souls and make us stronger. By having to work on healing our soul wounds and releasing the pain, we help ourselves to grow. Our consciousness develops and strengthens, which is what being alive is all about.

Ravensara helps us to heal these wounds gently. It resonates with the energy of the pain within the soul, and is powerful yet nurturing in its releasing and shedding of both remembered and unconscious trauma.

Botanical Information

Ravensara aromatica, whose traditional name is 'leaves that heal', is a magnificent, highly aromatic tree that grows chiefly in Madagascar. It grows to a height of 20 metres (66 feet) in humid, evergreen forests and bears fragrant leaves, bark and nuts, which exude a delicious spicy smell that's reminiscent of eucalyptus.

Ravensara essential oil is steam distilled from the leaves. Be careful not to confuse it with Ravensara bark, also called havozo, which is another essential oil made from the same tree. It has different properties because it's distilled from the bark, not the leaves.

Ravensara's Legendary Power

Madagascan mythology is full of stories about working with sacred plants. However, very little has been written down because these rich and colourful myths, known as *anganos*, are part of an oral tradition, held within the local communities.

In their traditional stories, the Madagascans worshipped a god called Zanahary. He created the world, as well as heaven and Earth. His son, Andrianerinerina, was made ruler of heaven. Andriamanitra (whose name means 'Fragrant Lord') was the third god in the trinity and reigned over the beloved ancestors who had great influence over the spiritual lives of the people.

Ravensara's Esoteric Qualities

This is a truly powerful oil, with the ability to release emotional blockages that are covering deeper soul wounds. We all have our own personal demons, which are often challenges presented to us as tools for growth. When we overcome and face them, we have the opportunity to spread our wings to receive more wisdom and light.

With the help of Ravensara, we can heal our soul wounds. They may have come from experiences in this lifetime or possibly be carried through from previous lives. They don't respond to drugs or even to talking therapies. This is because counselling and psychotherapy rarely get to the bottom of a deeply entrenched soul wound. The healing has to come from within and at a soul level.

Soul wounds manifest in many ways, presenting as troublesome feelings such as anxiety, fear, lack of self-worth, and an inability to accept and receive love. There's a general feeling that we're not deserving of all that's 'good' in life, leading to a heavy emptiness of heart.

Ravensara can perform very deep work, yet in a very gentle way, instilling the sense that we won't be given anything in our healing journey that we can't cope with. We simply have to trust the process.

When to Use Ravensara

Use Ravensara for soothing painful feelings that have a history. Soul wounds are the red buttons in our lives that flare up, especially when we're going through challenging times. They have a bearing on almost everything we feel and affect how we respond to events in our daily lives. They can have a big impact on our personal relationships and influence how we relate to the world.

Complex and hard to unravel, soul wounds can be the foundation of apparently groundless fears and phobias. Fear of spiders, snakes and heights, claustrophobia and agoraphobia can often be traced back to an event that pierced the soul, leaving a psychic splinter that festers. I like to think that Ravensara is the kindly pair of hands that removes the splinter so delicately and gently that all traces of it are gone and healing can begin.

Karmic Roots

Ravensara is governed by Neptune (*see page 149*) and has an affinity with Chiron.

Our soul wounds are tools for us to develop compassion for other beings and the archetypal energy of Chiron working through Ravensara shows us how to do this.

Discovered in 1977, Chiron is an asteroid lying between the orbits of Jupiter and Uranus. It was named after Chiron the centaur (half-man, half-horse), who was the immortal son of Cronus (known to the Romans as Saturn). Unlike almost all other centaurs, who were coarse and wild, Chiron was gentle, humane and skilled in healing. He's the archetype of the wounded healer, gravely injured after being accidentally shot by an arrow tipped with the Hydra's terrible venom. Being immortal meant that he couldn't die. Eventually, Prometheus changed places with Chiron, so that the centaur could finally escape from his agony. To honour him and give him a different sort of immortality, Zeus – the supreme god of the Greeks – placed him in the sky in the constellation of Sagittarius.

Guided Meditation

You might like to record this meditation before meditating with Ravensara. This will enable you to relax and listen to the meditation without unnecessary distractions. Simply follow the instructions for preparing yourself for a guided meditation (*see page 35*).

I'm here to heal your soul. These wounds don't respond to medicine or other treatments. They're the deep splinters at the very heart of you that are carried as a burden throughout life.

Open your heart. How does this feel? Fear, betrayal, abandonment, or being born in the wrong body, country, race or time can all be wounds in the soul.

Whatever you're feeling now, allow the deep, loving energy that I bring to pour like light through your soul and spirit. As you work with me, you may feel yourself gently rocking and swaying and spinning as your pain unravels.

Swaying, pulsations, rocking and undulations are always the motions felt as your body finds balance and comes back into its centre of stillness.

Flow with the movement. See yourself moving easily and gracefully out of the dissonant space. Whatever caused you to feel powerless or less than whole is now transmuting into a place of harmony and self-compassion.

Release the uneasy emotions. Float away from the negativity. This is simple and effortless when you focus with this intention.

Breathe again. Feel the comfort and openness of your physical being. Feel the freedom of internal movement and your connectedness to the rhythms of the Earth. You're at one with the dance of the cosmos. Give in and dance with the galactic flow. Stay in meditation and feel yourself dancing on the higher planes.

When you feel ready, slowly begin to come out of your meditation and float your energetic body back into your physical one. Keep the idea of internal sway as you wiggle your fingers and toes to remind your body of its extremities. Roll your head gently from side to side and enjoy the ease of movement. Slowly open your eyes to let in light and see your present surroundings. Smile and stretch your body in easy, fluid movements. Come fully back to the present.

This is my gift to you and also your gift to yourself. Your deep wounds will begin to heal now.

Ravensara's Key Points

◇   Releases inner pain and turmoil

◇   Repairs deep soul wounds

◇   Heals a sense of not being good enough

◇   Heals a sense of not being heard

◇   Eases gender issues or a sense of being in the wrong body

◇   Heals a feeling of being unloved or unlovable

◇   Soothes a sense of being abandoned

◇   Scent – spicy

◇   Affinity with the crown chakra

Contraindications

Not to be used during pregnancy.

CASE STUDY

Anyone seeing Polly would have thought that she had everything. She was a successful businesswoman at the top of her game, running a busy international sportswear company. Yet, she had a phobia that stopped her flying as high as she'd have liked.

She was actually afraid of flying, because she had claustrophobia. It prevented her from using lifts and underground trains, as well as planes. Even locking the lavatory door when she was in unfamiliar surroundings was a challenge.

Polly had tried hypnotherapy and homeopathy, but nothing had touched the root of the problem. The more successful she became, the worse her claustrophobia seemed to get. She couldn't understand why she felt like this.

When patients have a problem with no obvious cause, I take the intuitive route and invite them to take their time smelling the aromas of four different oils to see if any of them make an impression. I encourage them to take off their 'thinking heads', park their rational minds and let their hearts do the talking. Their impressions from smelling the oils could be a subtle sense of curiosity, a dazzling flash of intuition or a memory trawled up from long ago. We just need to be open to the experience and see what comes up.

Polly was drawn to Rose first, then to Patchouli, then Peru balsam and finally to Ravensara. She sat with the Ravensara bottle for a long time before closing her eyes and sharing a memory that rose from the depths of her early childhood. Polly confided that her mother sometimes locked her in a cupboard when she was a young child, while her mother went out shopping, often for hours on end. She came from an affluent family, who were outwardly very sociable and charming, but even as a child, Polly knew that her mother's behaviour towards her wasn't normal. She'd buried it and she'd never shared her 'dark' secret with anyone in case it caused trouble. Her parents divorced when she was eight and she was brought up by her grandmother, who told her to put all of her childhood terrors behind her.

In remembering her experiences Polly was able to release them, seeing them for what they were. She did a lot of work on forgiveness. Now, she's truly able to spread her wings and expand her business without being held back by her soul wound.

. . . .

Rose

Love and Learning to Love Yourself
and Your Inner Child

'Rose can be used to bring our consciousness closer to our angels, and to the angelic self that dwells within us. To inhale rose is to inhale the love and kisses of angels.'

VALERIE ANN WORWOOD, *AROMATHERAPY FOR THE SOUL*

Rose is the queen of oils – a veritable blessing in a bottle. This is the oil to use when unconditional love, divine understanding and wisdom are required to heal a person or situation that feels desperate and hopeless.

The energy of Rose oil, which is linked to the Divine Feminine, is gentle but extremely strong. It's an oil of both spirit and soul. Rose oil opens hearts, as well as helping to process sorrow and grief. It also helps us to receive spiritual knowledge.

There are two types of Rose oil: Rose Otto and Rose Absolute. Rose Otto is produced using steam distillation, while Rose Absolute is produced using a solvent extraction method.

Both oils are beautifully fragrant, but the extraction method of Rose Absolute produces more oil and a stronger scent, so is mostly used by the perfume industry, while Rose Otto is mostly used in aromatherapy. The name 'Rose Otto' originates from the Persian term 'attar of roses' and dates as far back as the 17th century. It comes from the Persian *atar-gul*, which means 'essence of roses', and from the Arabic *utur*, meaning 'perfumes' or 'aromas'.

Botanical Information

For the production of Rose oil, two major species of rose are cultivated. *Rosa damascena*, the damask rose, is widely grown in Bulgaria, China, India, Iran, Pakistan, Russia, Turkey and Uzbekistan. *Rosa centifolia*, the cabbage rose, is more commonly grown in Egypt, France and Morocco. It takes 3,500 kilograms (just under 800 pounds) of flowers to produce 1 kilogram (2 pounds) of essential oil through distillation: one drop of the oil contains 60 rose flowers. Harvesting of the flowers is done by hand before sunrise and the flowers are distilled on the same day. As a result of the low content of oil in the rose blooms and the labour-intensive production process, Rose oil commands a very high price.

Rose's Legendary Power

Roses appear as symbols of miraculous love at work in the world in accounts from all of the major religions. In ancient mythology, roses symbolized eternal love in stories of how gods interacted with both human beings and each other. Pagans use roses as decorations to represent their hearts.

Muslims view roses as symbols of the human soul, so smelling the scent of roses reminds them of their spirituality. Hindus and Buddhists see roses and other flowers as expressions of spiritual joy. Christians regard roses as reminders of the Garden of Eden, a paradise in a world that reflected God's design before sin corrupted it.

Rose's Esoteric Qualities

Throughout history, there have been many miracles and angelic encounters involving roses. And many people believe that angels and other holy figures use the scent of a rose as a physical sign of their spiritual presence.

In Islam, the fragrance of a rose represents the sacredness of people's souls. If the scent of a rose permeates the air, yet no actual roses are nearby, it's a sign that God, or one of His angels, is sending a message supernaturally, through clairalience (clear smelling). Such messages are meant to give encouragement.

In Catholicism, the scent of roses is often called the 'odour of sanctity', because it indicates the presence of spiritual holiness.

Self-love and self-care are cornerstones in becoming aware of who we are. One of the most profound, beautiful and simple lessons that rose teaches us is how to connect with love. It frees us and lifts us into spiritual realms, so that we can liberate and transform our base energy with the spirit of joy. The etheric form of this oil transmutes our heart's energy.

When to Use Rose

Anyone seeking a blessing of peace, emotional support or spiritual attunement will benefit from Rose oil. Adults (and children old enough to understand what's taking place) who are suffering from a grave illness, have been involved in a serious accident or trauma, or who are facing surgery or major medical tests, will feel uplifted after using this oil. It's beneficial for the elderly, especially when they're extremely frail; for those living with chronic physical or mental weakness; and those in need of healing, comfort and love for any reason, especially as a result of grief.

Rose oil can also be used for self-questing, when asking oneself the following questions:

◊ Am I aware of my own power?

◊ Am I recognizing my fullest potential?

◊ Am I playing the role of victim or victor?

◊ Am I using my power for the good of all?

◊ Am I connecting to my higher source of energy?

◊ Am I focusing effectively and beneficially?

◊ What action can I take to move in a better direction?

◊ What resources are available to me and how do I tap into them?

Karmic Roots

Rose has karmic roots with Venus (*see page 149*), Lemuria (*see page 87*), and also with the Divine Feminine.

The mystery of the Divine Feminine centres on the creative and nurturing aspects of Creation. The qualities of the Divine Feminine are love, peace, inspiration, healing, compassion, insight and wisdom. The Divine Feminine works with the Sacred Masculine to keep the universe in balance.

Guided Meditation

You might like to record this meditation before meditating with Rose oil. This will enable you to relax and listen to the meditation without unnecessary distractions. Simply follow the instructions for preparing yourself for a guided meditation (*see page 35*).

As you attune your sensitivity to the loveliness and beauty of Rose oil, you'll begin to understand the divine energy of the cosmic mother, who radiates love to heal humankind.

To commune with me, be peaceful and focus on the stillness within the middle of a rose. Centre your awareness on your heart as a soft focal point for consciousness. Then, within your inner silence, you'll hear my words.

Remember that love is the law of the Divine. We're in existence so we can learn to love. You love that you may learn to live. This is the only lesson that's required of humankind.

Love knows no boundaries. Breathe in the scent of love through your heart, pulling down light from the spiritual realm and allowing it to fill your whole being.

The divine act of summoning love through this oil can be used to heal hearts and minds from the distant past, allowing you to become a conductor of energy for healing in both the present and the future. Our human hearts change vibration when we work with the energy of rose and this connection becomes a sacred act. Generate a wave of love and return it to the world.

We're all being asked to master our emotions, and to observe and be aware of our own reactions to conflict when they're triggered by difficult events. Through the waves of anger, rage, frustration, sadness, sorrow and tragedy, new opportunities are starting to emerge. Our deeply wounded and grief-stricken hearts can connect to a new level of love consciousness, with both each other and ourselves, that's now starting to emerge.

We're being given divine assistance for transformation of our shadow and inner child. We're also being given support to release us of the emotional bleeding that we carry around in our bodies, in our chakras and in our cellular memories. It's these that we project onto others in the outside world. If we don't see our own shadow then we're in denial.

Whether we choose to accept our shadow or remain in denial, we're all going through an alchemical process of some kind. To feel secure, we must honour our own truth and integrity by embracing our shadow and healing our inner child, for it's these two archetypes that make us who we are.

Embrace your shadow side. Love is the key to healing and we have to give that love to ourselves first.

Rose's Key Points

◊ Encourages self-love and self-acceptance

◊ Brings peace and spiritual attunement

◊ Gives mental, emotional and physical support

◊ Scent – rich, sweet, deeply fragrant

◊ Affinity with the sacral, solar plexus and heart chakras

Contraindications

Rose Otto is an emmenagogue (it can induce or help menstruation), so shouldn't be used during pregnancy.

CASE STUDY

Georgia had everything that anyone could buy – a beautiful house, an expensive car, three horses and a holiday home in France. So why did she feel empty and sad?

She came for guidance after being diagnosed with the autoimmune disease lupus. During the consultation, Georgia explained what it's really like to live with a chronic illness every day and the path it takes you on. She also talked about how much she's had to learn about adapting to her new needs.

'The physical side is challenging enough. But mentally and emotionally, it's devastating. Despite all of the comforts I have in life, I'm not sure where to turn. I'm not enjoying anything any more. I'm having to learn to live with the unknown, and the uncertainty of ill health, fear and pain.'

*As we worked through several sessions, I became aware of the
anger Georgia felt with herself for being ill. We began to unpick
where this was coming from. This is what she told me:*

*'It got me questioning whether or not it was karmic in nature and
if it could be reversed. My mother hoped I'd follow in her footsteps
and become a doctor, but I just couldn't face all the hard work and
study. She told me once, in a fit of anger, that she could never love
me as much as my brother (who'd become a doctor) and that I was
a disappointment to her.*

*'I knew that I'd let her down, but hearing this made me feel that
I'd let myself down, too, by not living up to her expectations. I
began to loathe myself and the choices I'd made so I could lead a
glamorous, perhaps rather self-centred, life.'*

This seemed to be at the heart of her feelings about herself.

*Georgia began to work with Rose oil, meditating with it every
morning and evening, using positive affirmations about being
kinder to herself. After a month, she emailed and said she felt like
a new person. She'd even given herself permission to have a year
off from work (and not feel guilty about it). This came with the
realization that her illness had given her a purpose and a chance to
see both herself and her needs in a more loving and positive way.*

*'I now wonder if all illness and disease is a gift and a mystery
to serve my greatest and highest good. I had to feel the pain of*

envy about not being able to join in the fun and do the things spontaneously that most people take for granted. I had to feel the loneliness and isolation of not having a support network of friends around.

'Lupus taught me to be vulnerable – and to feel kinder to myself. And it taught me surrender, patience and acceptance. I'm feeling more at peace with life and grateful for the "good" moments during the day. Lupus has been a journey of initiation and awakening. And a lesson in learning that I need to love myself and heal my inner child. I suppose that we cannot truly love others until we've learned to love ourselves.'

. . . .

Sandalwood

Meditation and Listening Deeply

*'And listen deeply to what I am not telling you, for your heart
is eager to hear the mysteries that I speak from my soul.'*

ANONYMOUS

Sandalwood and its sacred service are all about deep listening.
We all like to think that we're good at listening, but it's
one of the hardest skills to master. We can learn professional
therapeutic listening, but there is of course another method
available to those of us with the sensitivity and patience to
practise it. This is the listening done with the heart, soul and
body. This is where sandalwood comes in.

Botanical Information

Sandalwood is a parasitic evergreen tree that's native to tropical
Asia. It grows up to 9 metres (30 feet) high and bears small pink-
purple flowers. There are several varieties of sandalwood tree, all

of which have to be decades old before chips made from their heartwood are aromatic enough to be steam distilled into oil. The source of the oil is primarily Indian sandalwood (*Santalum album*), Hawaiian sandalwood (*S. paniculatum*), Vanuatu sandalwood (*S. austrocaledonicum*) and Australian sandalwood (*S. spicatum*). True Indian sandalwood is now extremely rare and another species is usually substituted. The oil ranges between pale yellow and pale gold, with a warm, woody and exotic scent.

Sandalwood's Legendary Power

Sandalwood oil encourages stillness of the mind and a meditative state. It helps us to listen to inner wisdom from our higher selves. Sandalwood was mentioned in the Vedic scriptures of the 5th century BCE and had associations with embalming, as well as enhancing harmony, peace and serenity.

It's been used in rituals for thousands of years, including Buddhist and Muslim rituals. Buddhists believe that sandalwood is one of the sacred scents of the lotus, and can be used during meditation to calm and focus the mind. In Hindu rites, sandalwood paste is often used to cleanse ritual tools before ceremonies. In India, the wood is used for its talismanic powers in temple carvings, shrines and jewellery.

Modern paganism values sandalwood for space clearing and other forms of purification.

Sandalwood's Esoteric Qualities

Sandalwood's soothing, calming and grounding. It helps us to slow down the world around us when it feels fractious and stressful, giving us clarity when we find ourselves in muddled situations.

Esoterically, it can stabilize chaotic energy and pride, providing an etheric refuge from difficult external forces, such as negative energies and encroaching thought forms.

Sandalwood also opens our inner ears, enabling us to hear what isn't being said. In addition, sandalwood enables every aspect of ourselves – our heart, our body and our soul – to listen. This is the listening that senses a blockage of energy and intuitively moves our hands to a particular spot while we perform our gentle touch. It's the listening that gives us a gut feeling about what's required to best serve our friend when they're unable to tell us; the listening that's inexplicable but that gives us the knowledge we cannot receive through other means. This is the listening that goes beyond the physical, giving our work depth and its greatest meaning. This is the listening that comes from the stillness within ourselves, the 'knowing' that comes to us as we develop our connection with spirit, as well as the deeply profound soul-to-soul connection that we can sometimes be fortunate enough to establish with a friend.

Heart-based listening comes from holding someone's hand, making eye contact, being close to them, and opening our heart and soul to whatever they wish to share with us. This should be done with love, compassion and understanding, not only being aware of what they have said, but also what they haven't said. It's about respecting that sacred sharing. This very profound, deeply involved listening allows significant shifts to happen, and with these shifts come healing, acceptance and inner peace.

When to Use Sandalwood

Sandalwood oil soothes the restless spirit, bringing it peace and tranquillity. It hushes a busy mind by slowing down what can be an endless loop of anxious or obsessive thoughts, or endless overthinking.

Negative emotional states such as stress, anxiety, anger, rage, restlessness and nervousness can all be eased by Sandalwood. Even physical conditions, including insomnia, headaches and migraines, triggered by these emotional patterns can be alleviated.

Sandalwood's gentle otherworldly vibration calls us to prayer and helps us to connect with sacred spaces. It urges us to slow down, stop worrying and into tune in to love, beauty, harmony and the natural forces of the world.

Karmic Roots

Sandalwood has karmic connections with our own planet, Earth (*see page* 78).

Guided Meditation

You might like to record this meditation before meditating with Sandalwood oil. This will enable you to relax and listen to the meditation without unnecessary distractions. Simply follow the instructions for preparing yourself for a guided meditation (*see page* 35).

When we truly allow ourselves to experience the connection we have with Mother Earth, and with our own intuition, we create abundance and radiance in our lives. Take a moment to reflect on the love that surrounds you and build on this energy to create even more nurturing love in your life. Know that love is limitless.

Step out of the noise around you and sit within the silence of the universe to hear the most profound teachings of all. We can only fill our souls when we're still enough to listen. Hear without feeling overwhelmed or challenged by restlessness. The messenger comes from a distant place to show us the real thresholds that we need to cross.

Find ways to support dialogue and open communication, creating a space to express your feelings openly. We're all being rewired for a

new level of consciousness. Many traumatic things are happening
in the outer world that may trigger our primal fears about survival
and vulnerability, yet people are instinctively finding the courage to
rise up in their own way to help others in need and to change the
status quo. But, first, you have to slow down and listen.

Sandalwood's Key Points

◊ Encourages listening with the heart

◊ Quietens mental anguish

◊ Soothes mental chatter

◊ Grounds and stabilizes

◊ Affinity with the sacral and crown chakras

Contraindications

◊ Women who are breastfeeding and young children shouldn't use this oil.

◊ Care should be taken by people with liver disease or cancer.

CASE STUDY

Stan was a very successful therapist with lots of clients and a long
waiting list. He'd always loved his profession, but he confided that

he was feeling stale and not enjoying the stories he heard any more. This used to be his favourite part of his work, his real calling, and he'd always thought of himself as a good listener, but he realized that for some reason, unknown to him, he wasn't a good listener any longer. So, what was this all about?

Stan realized that he'd stopped really listening and so had stopped hearing other people at a deep level. He explained that he secretly felt 'full up' with hearing about other people's traumas and they seemed to be affecting his own wellbeing. This brought him a feeling of guilt.

'I realize that I'm still trying to hold the space for my clients and listen on some sort of adequate level, but I'm not actually giving them my full attention.

'And so my own preconceptions, judgements, preoccupations, personal concerns and anxieties are colouring my response to them. This means I'm not being a good therapist to them,' he explained.

As a way of beginning to help him, I suggested that he go on a silent retreat, where he could 'listen' to himself and not the words of others. This way, he'd have the chance of connecting with a sacred oil, as well as receive teaching from it through meditation and reflection. After feeling an instant connection with it, he chose Sandalwood.

Stan wrote to me a few weeks later, saying, 'Through meditation with the oil, I can come into presence in my body and give myself fully to the words spoken by the oil. It guided me to look again at how I was listening and urged me to "hear" without the pressure of having to give a trained, boundaried and calculated professional response.

'Instead, I could allow myself to respond as another human being. I'm now trying to hear with my heart. I'm open to hear what they say, bringing compassion and my full attention to them. If I'm moved to tears, so be it, I can cry with them. If I'm brought to laughter then I'll laugh with them. This new way of listening is changing my work as a therapist. I'll now engage more and from a deeper place of connection.

'I realized, how could I carry out my work with integrity if I didn't listen with my heart? To listen to a client's pain and anguish, to accept it, to witness it, and to allow the profound and deeply moving to surface is one of the greatest gifts I can probably offer as a therapist. It's a privilege to be trusted by my clients and to serve them in such a humbling way.'

Listening is one of the most valuable things we can do for other people but, sadly, it's a skill that's often neglected or not done properly, if at all. Many of us lead busy lives and don't seem to have the time to give someone our full attention or make a conscious effort to engage with what we're being told.

From the myrrhophore's perspective, by honouring this, we help to create the sacred. If we can embody all that we've been taught through the ages, through the long lineage of wise women and priestesses who have gone before us, listening to the troubled and the sick, then we've earned our privilege in working with the souls of those who have come to us for help.

. . . .

Silver Fir

Journeying and Accessing Personal Power

*'Look at every path closely and deliberately, then ask ourselves
this crucial question: Does the path have a heart? If it does,
then the path is good. If it doesn't, then it is of no use to us.'*
CARLOS CASTENADA, *THE TEACHINGS OF DON JUAN*

The first time I worked with this oil I was catapulted
back into a past life as a nomadic medicine woman in
Siberia. Trudging through the snow, dressed in wraps and furs,
carrying a heavy bag of skin and wood, I smelled the intense
menthol-like crisp air in the forests. In the inky sky was a huge
Full Moon and twinkling stars. Wolves were howling in the
distance. In that intense flashback I reconnected with forest
medicine and the power of the trees around me. Breathing into
that bottle of Silver Fir oil with my eyes closed and my heart
open reminded me of being free and wild. I felt very sure of the
path I followed.

The energy of this oil is all about breaking out, being released and shaking off the shackles. It demands that you step into your power and fill the space destined for you.

Its message is 'Be bigger than you even dare.' Life is an invitation to dance, so spread your eagle wings, own your power and fly.

Even now, when I work with this oil, I can hear my ancestors talking to me and encouraging me to make my way through the forest. It's a magnificent oil for spiritual questing, meeting ancestors, and connecting with wisdom keepers and ancestral memory.

Botanical Information

Silver Fir oil is obtained by steam distilling the glossy green needles of the silver fir (*Abies alba*). The tree, which is evergreen, is grown commercially for its timber and also as Christmas trees (although other species have replaced it to a great extent). It's a native of the mountains of Northern Europe. A mature silver fir can reach to over 50 metres (164 feet) tall.

Silver Fir's Legendary Power

The fir tree appears in several myths. Followers of Dionysus, the Greek god of wine and intoxication (who was Bacchus to the Romans), would worship him in the woods rather than in temples. Maenads, or wild women, accompanied him on his travels around the world, carrying staffs whose tips were decorated with pine cones. Cybele (also known as Kybele) was the mother goddess of Anatolia. A sacred silver fir, specially decorated, was always at the centre of her mountain orgies. One of the myths about her claims that her beloved consort, Attis, killed himself at the foot of a pine tree and was transformed into a pine tree. The pre-Hellenic goddess of childbirth was Eileithyia and the gum of the silver fir was sometimes called the menses of Eileithyia, suggesting that it had medicinal uses in childbirth.

The Northwestern tribes of Native Americans, and especially in the area that's now Washington State, used fir cones for weather magic. Members of the Haisla people in what is now British Columbia would blacken their faces with pitch made from the silver fir tree as a sign of mourning.

Silver Fir's Esoteric Qualities

Plato wrote that the silver fir could help in divination. It's certainly a valuable oil both for initiation rites, and for when we want to explore the labyrinth of the human mind and the imagination. If something is hidden or suppressed, Silver Fir oil will bring it out of the shadows. It can also be used when we're questing for personal power and revelation.

Silver fir has an affinity with the mystery of life itself. It gives us the courage to become at one with the wild, thereby strengthening our intuition and survival skills. With its help, we can experience the energy of the deep, mysterious forest and the wilderness that lies beyond. It strengthens and enriches our connection with nature and the creatures that inhabit it, whether they're seen or unseen.

When to Use Silver Fir

This oil helps us when we need to grow and develop, when we know that our current path is too restricting or our way of life is no longer fulfilling. It gives us the intuition to find a new direction in life. It can also help us when we want to be released from tight inner boundaries that, instead of anchoring and stabilizing us, are holding us in a prison of our own making.

Karmic Roots

Silver fir has karmic links with the Earth (*see page 78*).

Guided Meditation

You might like to record this meditation before meditating with Silver Fir. This will enable you to relax and listen to the meditation without unnecessary distractions. Simply follow the instructions for preparing yourself for a guided meditation (*see page 35*).

I'm anchored in the ground yet, with my crown in heaven, I draw in the verdant, abundant forest filled with colour and sound.

Sense the energy rising through my branches, releasing any blockages that are stopping you from growing, and draw down light into your roots. Express your vitality. Feel the heaviness in your soul lighten and dissolve.

Remember that your limits are self-imposed, reflecting your limited view of yourself. Come out of the darkness and enter the light. Smell the earth, hear the birdsong and allow all of your senses to expand.

I ask you to stand in your own power. Release yourself from self-imposed obligations. Know that you're a beloved child of the forest and in service to those around you. I'll help you to see wider and further than you ever imagined.

I'll attune you to the frequencies of the universe. All you have to do is allow this to happen and the effect can be instantaneous.

Silver Fir's Key Points

◊ Helps us to discover our personal power

◊ Enables us to find a new direction in life

◊ Provides release from outworn patterns

◊ Gives the courage to be ourselves

◊ Scent – fresh, dry and coniferous like a forest

◊ Affinity with the brow chakra

Contraindications

Oils from a variety of fir trees are sold as fir needle oil, so it's important to confirm that you're buying oil made from *Abies alba* and not a different species.

CASE STUDY

Alfie lived in a small flat in Manchester. Although he'd left university with a good degree in engineering, he'd found life increasingly tough ever since. He'd applied for lots of jobs but still hadn't found one. Gradually, his confidence had ebbed away until he started going out less and less. His friendships had faded and he was becoming fearful about leaving the flat.

I visited him and found a pale young man whose life was getting smaller as the four walls around him closed in. His world was shrinking and his energy was restricted. He was hemmed in and depressed.

Alfie told me that he spent a lot of time thinking about his teenage years, which had been sociable and active. He'd been a member of an athletics club and loved being outside. Now, he couldn't even put on a pair of shoes without feeling a sense of dread.

I asked him, gently, if he could turn his thoughts from contemplation to meditation. I sensed that his deeper self was ready to blossom but he needed a trigger for this to happen.

He then told me about his special place as a child living on the edge of a forest. Whenever he could, he'd play among the trees, even though he played alone. He felt that the trees communicated with him.

Silver Fir oil carries the inner radiance of the trees. It's an energy of expansion and helps to stretch the aura when it's used in meditation. I blended a vial of oil designed to help Alfie's leaves to unfurl. The oil made him dream and this is what he told me:

'Some kind of ancient spirit came through the crackling leaves. I smelled the soil and heard rustling branches brushing against me. I looked up to see towering firs pointing up, touching the sky. The trees spoke and I felt from them not only a sense of respect and sympathy, but also encouragement to keep walking. I was in a space like a green cathedral and the trees created a mass energy field that moved through me, lifting my own vibration. The trees said they'd stand beside me if I could get into the open.'

One Saturday, Alfie asked his mum to drive him to the New Forest in the South of England, where they spent the weekend *camping and walking. Alfie began to feel stronger and within six months, he'd found a job as a gardener in a cottage surrounded by fir trees. The oil brought him back into harmony again and literally helped him to turn over a new leaf.*

. . . .

Spikenard

The Consolamentum Oil – a Glimpse of Paradise

'Then Mary took pound of ointment of spikenard,
very costly, and anointed the feet of Jesus.'
JOHN 12:3

Spikenard is a most ancient and powerful oil, with a long lineage that connects it with ancient Egyptian and Babylonian temple traditions. Later, the Essene and Cathar communities also worked with it for holy and healing purposes. In those days, it was one of the most valued essential oils and extremely expensive.

Botanical Information

Spikenard (*Nardostachys jatamansi*) belongs to the valerian family. It's a native of the Himalayas, growing to about 1 metre (3 feet) high and bearing pink flowers. But it's the rhizome that's steam distilled to make Spikenard essential oil. Sadly, spikenard is such a valuable plant commercially that it's now considered to be critically endangered and is on the International Union for Conservation of Nature (IUCN) Red List of Threatened Species. It shouldn't be confused with spike lavender (*Lavandula latifolia*), which is a completely different plant.

The oil is pale yellow to amber, with a heavy, deep and spicy scent that not everyone likes.

Spikenard's Legendary Power

One of the most memorable stories about spikenard involves Mary Magdalene anointing Jesus's feet with it at the Last Supper. The disciples criticized her – a jar of spikenard, or 'nard', as it was called, was so expensive that the quantity she used could have probably kept a family in food and drink for an entire year.

Within the myrrhophore tradition, Mary was known to be a highly trained priestess and an expert in energy healing. In particular, she was skilled in the art of aiding transition from this world to the next. She knew exactly what she was doing with her jar of spikenard, which was the main oil for transition 2,000 years ago. It resonated with the energy of death and transition, and was used esoterically to ease the passage of the dying by preparing the spirit and soul.

Some say that spikenard enables the body to open up to the Holy Spirit. Certainly this was the view of the Cathars, a religious sect with whom Jesus is reputed to have spent time as a young man. The Cathars were well known for both their healing abilities and their simple, pure way of living.

After the Crucifixion, the Cathars believed that they held the knowledge of Jesus's inner and most secret teachings, which maintained that the Holy Spirit's power could be passed on by direct transmission through the laying on of hands. When we receive this gift of the spirit, which flows through the hands like a divine current, we have a direct link to Jesus. Spikenard was used in the initiation and transmission process, probably as a result of anointing and by energetically opening the portal through which the Holy Spirit could pass.

The Cathars were both renowned and envied for the power this gave them. They used it to perform an extraordinary spiritual baptism called the Consolamentum. This was given to the sick or dying, with the power to show loved ones and the dying a glimpse of Paradise. It might only be for a brief moment, but it was just long enough to experience the dazzling light and overpowering love that lay beyond the threshold. When people saw this radiance and felt the energy of Paradise, their fear of death was removed. This is why the baptism was called the Consolamentum or solace baptism.

The Consolamentum has a great affinity with women healers. In Cathar times, the women of the sect were known to travel about, teaching the mysteries of the soul and healing the sick.

Spikenard's Esoteric Qualities

This oil leads us across the sacred threshold to be with those we've loved and who are now in spirit. It opens the heart to receive the gifts of the spirit and the mysteries of the soul. It holds the key to the religious rite known as the Consolamentum, which was known to elected priests and initiates of the Cathar sect.

The original Cathar movement was revived between the 12th and 14th centuries, especially in what's now Northern Italy and Southern France. However, these men and women were massacred for not wanting to pass on their most precious skill of offering the dying person a brief experience of Paradise. The vision and knowledge that came with this was such an enormous psychic event that, having experienced it, one would never fear death again.

This rite has been kept alive by the 'few' and is still passed on in the traditional way by the laying on of hands.

When to Use Spikenard

As the Cathars showed, Spikenard is a very valuable oil for use during the dying process. It can also be used by those who are bereaved and who are longing for comfort and insight into the mysteries of death.

Additionally, it's an oil for people who accord with the priestly archetypes, either in this life or carried over from a past life. It can be used when someone needs access to hermetic knowledge, but only after pledging allegiance to the guardian deity Hermes Trismegistus.

Spikenard helps individuals who are using love to change their vibrational level to the frequency of Christ Consciousness and unconditional love, so they can access the deeper chambers of the etheric heart.

Karmic Roots

Spikenard has karmic links with Arcturus and the Great White Brotherhood.

Arcturus is the brightest star in the constellation Boötes and is the fourth brightest star in the northern hemisphere. It's an orange giant and lies 36 light years from Earth. Esoteric knowledge teaches us that Arcturus is populated by human-like beings who are working together to form a group consciousness. They're powerful healers but work with many other spiritual energies, as well.

Also known as the Ascended Masters, the Great White Brotherhood is a group of immensely enlightened and powerful immortal souls whose purpose is to make every human aware of their divine nature. Many mystery schools have been developed on Earth in order to spread this teaching while avoiding the persecution that inevitably followed whenever it became public. Members of the Great White Brotherhood include such teachers as Jesus Christ and Buddha.

Guided Meditation

You might like to record this meditation before meditating with Spikenard. This will enable you to relax and listen to the meditation without unnecessary distractions. Simply follow the instructions for preparing yourself for a guided meditation (*see page 35*).

> *I'll console you and lead you across the sacred threshold to be with those you've loved and who now live in spirit.*
>
> *By parting the veils of this world, I'll show you the glory of living in spirit and help you to connect with the souls of those who have transitioned. I'm the Consolamentum.*
>
> *I open a space within your heart, so that you can receive the mysteries. You'll become a channel for divine energies and light will flow through your hands to reach across the sacred threshold.*
>
> *I invite you to call each of your loved ones and ask them to stand with you. They bring gifts of the spirit.*

As you listen to me, which parts of your body's energies are open and receptive, and which are closed and repelling my message? (You should pause here to check your body's sensations.) Do these parts of your body have a message for you? (Pause and listen for a message to come to you.)

Your inner knowing reminds you that you've chosen your loved ones for a karmic purpose. They're here as a reflection of something within yourself. When you look at them, you're looking in a mirror showing your history, your ancestry and your patterning.

Allow your inner understanding to receive the message that your loved ones have for you today. Be aware of a softening in your being. Feel a sense of forgiveness and love, bringing you to a deeper level of compassion towards your loved ones in spirit.

Can you flow with the tides and currents of the universal ocean? Can you allow yourself to rock gently in the rhythm of the universal waves as they wash around you? (Pause... here.) I, Spikenard, am the key to being in the flow of the celestial sea and am the door to Paradise.

Spikenard's Key Points

◊ Removes fear of the dying process

◊ Brings comfort to the bereaved

◊ Teaches us to work with the complex gateways of the psyche and the gateway to Paradise

◊ Opens the heart

◊ Scent – deep, heavy and spicy

◊ Affinity with the heart chakra

Contraindications

None known.

CASE STUDY

Freda is a nurse and was the carer for George, an elderly retired priest suffering from Alzheimer's disease. As he became less able to talk and communicate, Freda and her family tried to find other ways to get him to respond.

Freda brought in CDs to play at his bedside and also a wooden stringed sounding bowl, which he plucked every now and then and seemed to enjoy. However, George was progressively 'slipping from view', as Freda put it, and sinking into a space where no one could reach him.

George's daughter, Sarah, visited him often but was increasingly sad that she could no longer make a connection with him. She explained, 'It's as if he's left home and his body's empty and

surviving without his spirit being present.' There seemed no way of reaching him any more.

Having attended one of my sacred oils workshops, Freda decided to start massaging the soles of George's feet to try to stimulate some interest in him and see if she could shift his energy, which felt stuck and sticky. Freda remembered that the soles of the feet have a connection with the soul and chose to work with Spikenard, knowing that the oil has an affinity with priestly archetypes.

After several weeks, George began to sing quietly. Sarah heard about this and asked if she could massage his feet, too. Spikenard's pungent, spicy smell was pleasant and Sarah greatly enjoyed rubbing the oil into her father's feet as a way of showing her love for him.

One night, having massaged George's feet shortly before she helped to settle him for the evening, Sarah drove home and fell asleep in front of the television. When she woke, she was aware of having dreamed that George had appeared to her, many years younger than he was now. He was reunited with her mother, who'd died five years earlier.

George told Sarah that she mustn't worry, because he was now living in a beautiful place and his body (in the care home) didn't house his spirit any more. He said she mustn't mourn that he'd be leaving his earthly life soon. Instead, he asked her to celebrate

225

everything that was so good for him. He stated that he was able to live in two worlds until the time was right for him to pass on.

He lived for a few more weeks and when he died, Sarah knew that he was happy and in the right place, and at the right time.

. . . .

Violet Leaf

Extreme Grief

*'The reason it hurts so much to separate is because our souls
are connected. Maybe they always have been and will be.'*
NICHOLAS SPARKS, *THE NOTEBOOK*

This is a wondrous cure. Violet flowers are so delicate and small, yet their gift is so powerful. It's strange that Violet oil and Violet Leaf oil (which is an absolute and is much easier to obtain) are so little recognized. The violet is an unsung hero of the plant world but holds the key to healing hearts and souls consumed with grief – a problem carried by so many.

I often recommend Violet oil (which I make myself) to care homes, especially those caring for patients with dementia. Many of these patients are holding on to a pattern of trauma, which they're unable to put into words. If Violet oil cannot be obtained, Violet Leaf oil works almost as well. It gently releases the grief, laying it to rest and healing the wounds that lie beneath.

Botanical Information

As its name suggests, Violet Leaf oil is made from the leaves of *Viola odorata*. The violet is a small perennial plant with heart-shaped dark green leaves and small, fragrant flowers on delicate stems. The flowers can be white, blue, violet or deep purple. It's native to Europe and Asia, and is grown commercially in France for use in the perfume industry. Violet Leaf oil has a strong leafy scent and a floral undertone.

Violet's Legendary Power

For the ancient Greeks, the violet was a symbol of fertility and love, so was a prime ingredient in love potions. It also became the symbol of Athens and the city was described as *iostephanos*, meaning 'crowned with violets'. The Greek myth of Cybele and Attis recounts that a carpet of violets sprang up where Attis's blood was shed after he killed himself.

Ancient Britons steeped the flowers in goat's milk and used them as a cosmetic. In medieval times, the violet was found in most monastery gardens throughout Europe, where it was grown as a cure for melancholy.

It was traditionally thought that carrying violets kept evil spirits at bay and that a tisane made from violets would mend a broken heart. Violets placed under a pillow were said to give prophetic dreams.

Violet's Esoteric Qualities

Like the colour from which it takes its name, Violet Leaf oil carries an extremely high frequency. Its luminous, radiant energy bathes and feeds the aura. The colour violet has the fastest vibrational frequency and the shortest wavelength in the entire spectrum. This quality combines with the vibrational signature of the essential oil to create a very strong, dynamic and profound healing tool. Violet Leaf wraps a powerful and protective cloak around us when we need healing.

Violet works with the crown chakra, with a powerful influence on the brain and nervous system. It's a purifying force and stimulates spiritual perception.

Of all of the oils and absolutes, this is the one that seems to contain an otherworldly quality, which I think is handed down through the planes by the fairy realms. Don't be deceived by its aroma, which is fresh, green and not particularly memorable. Violet Leaf is like an atomic medicine for the soul.

When to Use Violet Leaf

When someone is experiencing such extreme grief that they're inconsolable, Violet Leaf will give them comfort and strengthen their heart, so they can move through this stage into a state of acceptance. This is also an oil to use for anyone dealing with the death of someone young and who might not have been expected to die so soon. Traumatic experiences in early childhood can also be healed with Violet Leaf. It has an affinity with the wistfulness and longing that can come with wishing that the past had been different and happier.

Violet Leaf oil can also be used when someone is struggling with anxiety, or even despair, and doesn't know how to cope, having reached the end of their tether. In addition, it can be used for tension or when someone is affected by sudden exhaustion.

Karmic Roots

Violet Leaf is connected with the planet Venus (*see page 149*) at a karmic level.

Guided Meditation

You might like to record this meditation before meditating with Violet Leaf. This will enable you to relax and listen to the meditation without unnecessary distractions. Simply follow the instructions for preparing yourself for a guided meditation (*see page 35*).

> *Call on me when the pain of deep grief is unrelenting, when the crying and the state of missing a beloved has become a deep, raw wound that nothing seems to heal.*

I'm gentle but strong. I'll release you from the deepest pain of your soul's suffering. Even holding a bottle containing a few precious drops of my essence may bring a soothing shift in your heart. You'll heal and greet joy in your life once more. I've a soothing and high vibration. I'm a powerful gift from the Earth that will hold your soul in a place of total love and release.

Note: seeing colours during a violet meditation is a common and healing experience in itself. According to Ayurveda and other Eastern healing systems, seeing any colour that relates to a specific chakra or energy centre in the body means that healing is taking place in that area of the body. Seeing violet can be a sign of the deep healing taking place within the soul.

Violet Leaf's Key Points

◊ For intractable grief and despair

◊ For coming to terms with the death of children and young people

◊ Brings comfort and strength

◊ Scent – woody with floral undertones

◊ Affinity with the crown chakra

Contraindications

It can cause sensitivity in some people, so should be used with caution at first.

CASE STUDY

Anya was referred to me by a close friend. Her only son, Niall, had died six years before in a snowboarding accident, when he was 27.

She was so racked with grief that she felt as though she'd died with him. Although she was gradually beginning to pick up the threads of her own life again, Anya still wasn't able to clear out Niall's room, so it was exactly as he'd left it. She now has grandchildren, by her daughter, and Niall's room would have been an ideal bedroom for them when they come to stay if Anya had been able to empty it of his possessions.

Anya told me about her continuing links with Niall. 'I talk to my son in my head. I lie on his bed sometimes during the day, ask him what he's doing. Sometimes I ask his advice. I even send texts to his mobile phone. Sometimes I shout at him. I'd like to be able to remember all of the special things we did together, but I'm too upset and, anyway, my memory is somehow blocked. Life is moving on around me and I've two beautiful grandsons who are always talking about Uncle Niall. I want to have a bigger space for them in my heart, but so much of my energy is taken up with grieving. What can I do?'

We talked at length and also spoke to Niall's spirit, which seemed to be with us. Anya told him that she'd always love him but that she needed to live her life again. I suggested that she meditated after placing a few drops of Violet Leaf on the skin above her heart chakra at night.

Although Anya was still holding Niall's memory close to her heart, she decided to begin making changes in his room. After some weeks, Anya made a memory box for Niall's belongings and began recording memories about him in a small book that she wanted her family to read. The memory box contains photographs, drawings, favourite songs, stories and little objects, including his comb and a scarf that still smells of him. She has plans to repaint his room and put in bunk beds for her two grandsons.

In addition, she plans to create a Facebook page for mothers who have lost sons, as a way of celebrating their lives.

Anya is slowly reclaiming her life. She explained, 'I felt surprised, moved and challenged by working with Violet Leaf oil, but it was worth it because I can begin to feel alive again.'

Yarrow

Sensitivity, Fear and Soul Wounds

*'Sensitive people should be treasured. They love deeply and
think deeply about life. They are loyal, honest and true.
The simple things sometimes mean the most to them. They
don't need to change – their purity makes them who they are.'*

ANONYMOUS

Yarrow has been a companion plant for us for centuries.
Its oil is very potent in protecting people who are highly
sensitive to energy. It wraps a gentle cloak of protection around
us when we need it, enabling us to keep our energies distinct
from those of the people and places we encounter. It stops us
from becoming like psychic blotting paper, soaking up other
people's emotions, sometimes without even being aware of it
until we realize that we feel drained, tearful or frightened but
cannot explain why. It also helps us to heal our soul wounds
– those raw, agonizing areas of our psyche that are like an
Achilles heel.

Botanical Information

Yarrow (*Achillea millefolium*) is a perennial herb that can grow to about 1 metre (3 feet) tall. It has woody stems, feathery green leaves and dense flat heads of pinky-white flowers. Yarrow is commonly found growing wild in Europe, North America and Western Asia, although many cultivars grow in gardens, too. The oil is steam distilled from dried yarrow plants.

Yarrow's Legendary Power

Yarrow has a long medicinal legacy that stretches back tens of thousands of years. When a grave that's more than 60,000 years old was excavated in Shanidar in Iran, it was found to contain pollen grains from eight medicinal plants, including yarrow. The plant treats fever, digestive ailments and respiratory infections, among other conditions.

Yarrow's medicinal qualities were known to the ancient Greeks and the plant gets part of its name from its association with the great hero Achilles, who is reputed to have used it to treat men who were injured in battle. Yarrow is known to stop bleeding.

The ancient Chinese were also familiar with yarrow's medicinal uses, especially for treating bites and other wounds. In addition, dried yarrow stalks were important, because a bundle of 50 stalks was used to cast the *I Ching* oracle. They were gradually superseded by three coins.

Yarrow is useful in other forms of divination, as well. Rubbing the plant on the eyelids was said to boost psychic abilities and yarrow tea can be drunk as a prelude to divination. Throwing yarrow plants across a threshold may stop negative spirits from crossing it.

Yarrow's Esoteric Qualities

Yarrow is an oil of great power and protection. It strengthens the aura and is especially good against psychic attack. This means it's excellent for emotional and highly sensitive people, as well as for empaths who absorb the pain of others, often to their own detriment because they cannot rid themselves of it easily. Yarrow oil also helps to guard against absorbing the energy of other people's diseases, especially when giving them healing or caring for them.

This is an oil with visionary qualities, so it can help us to see into the future. It also has the reputation for being able to awaken the psychic senses and perceptions. It can brighten dreams and is helpful for anyone wanting to practise lucid dreaming.

Telepathy can be developed over time with the aid of Yarrow oil. Adepts use it for levitation and it can bring conscious cooperation with occult forces.

When to Use Yarrow

Use Yarrow oil to strengthen your boundaries if you're extremely sensitive to the energies around you and tend to absorb them into your own energy field. This can apply to the energies from situations or people. Yarrow is therefore an oil to use whenever someone needs psychic protection. This is because it will form a barrier between them and outer influences. If we're ever troubled by a deep sense of fear, whether we know the reasons for it or not, Yarrow will help to ease our feelings and stabilize our emotions.

Sometimes when we're very open to the energy fields of other people, we're also extremely sensitive to electromagnetic frequencies, such as those emitted by mobile phones, Wi-Fi and computers. Yarrow will help to clear the effects of electromagnetic pollution.

Karmic Roots

Yarrow has karmic links with Neptune (*see page 149*).

Guided Meditation

You might like to record this meditation before meditating with Yarrow. This will enable you to relax and listen to the meditation without unnecessary distractions. Simply follow the instructions for preparing yourself for a guided meditation (*see page 35*).

Let me help you meditate on fear. Harness my essence for protection against negative influences.

The shape of each soul is different. When a spiritual situation is too intense and overwhelming, a sense of fear can hide the light from you.

The shadows can help you to befriend the darkness, gently illuminating the dark centres of the mind and the labyrinth of the soul. I'll help you, in the shadows, to be tender to your senses.

When your unconscious mind becomes illuminated, with me as your guide, the dark forces will no longer hold you. Stand in your power.

Yarrow's Key Points

◊ Provides psychic protection

◊ Strengthens the energy field

◊ Stabilizes the emotions

◊ Clears the effects of electromagnetic pollution

◊ Affinity with the base chakra

Contraindications

◊ Yarrow can cause skin irritation in sensitive people, so should always be mixed with a carrier oil before being applied to the skin.

◊ It can cause headaches, especially in people who are susceptible to them.

◊ Yarrow is an emmenagogue (it can induce or help menstruation), so shouldn't be used during pregnancy.

CASE STUDY

Angharad is a celebrant who takes many funerals. She's a very compassionate and caring woman, but also very sensitive.

Recently, she'd been helping a young couple who'd lost a baby at birth, born sleeping. She told me that she'd met the parents to help them to plan their baby's funeral and had become so distressed by their story that she'd found herself with tears rolling down her cheeks. The couple hadn't seemed to notice, but Angharad had been left with questions about how she'd reacted. If she could be so overwhelmed by emotion when talking to the bereaved, was her professionalism at stake?

'Am I in the wrong job? Shouldn't I just learn to swallow my feelings at the risk of closing down emotionally? I feel as if I need some sort of emotional buffer, especially when I'm working with grieving people,' she told me.

Angharad wondered whether or not I could recommend an oil that'd give her an emotional barrier while still enabling her to be empathetic and sensitive to other people's needs. We discussed Yarrow and its gift for strengthening energetic boundaries and emotions, and I gave her a vial of the oil.

Ever since our conversation, Angharad has used Yarrow in a simple ritual before doing any work as a celebrant. She washes, lights a candle and meditates on the task at hand. She puts a few drops of Yarrow on her heart and throat chakras to make her feel strong and able to hold the space. She told me what a difference it's made to her.

'What I do know is that shedding tears isn't a weakness. Nor is it unprofessional in my capacity as a celebrant; although I respect that some feel we must remain stoical.

'I've thought about this a lot and talked to other celebrants. It requires a certain professional strength to open our hearts in order to feel someone else's loss so deeply that we cannot walk away from the experience without being changed in some significant way.

'Using Yarrow has really liberated me and stopped me from feeling so bombarded by my emotions. I'm now able to turn down the volume of my feelings.'

Glossary of Terms

Abortifacient: chiefly said of a drug able to induce abortion, therefore best avoided during pregnancy.

Accidie: spiritual or mental sloth.

Alchemical: magical process of transformation and/or creation.

Anointing: when performed with a sacred oil, it is a ritualized blessing as well as a sacred and devotional act.

Caduceus: ancient Greek or Roman herald's wand, invariably with two serpents entwined round it, carried by the messenger god Hermes or Mercury.

Censer: vessel in which incense is burned during a religious ceremony.

Chemotype: an essential oil chemotype has differing therapeutic properties and is derived from a plant with the same visual appearance and characteristics, but with differing components chemically.

Clairalience: ability to receive psychic information through the subtle sense of smell.

Consolamentum: spiritual baptism given to the sick or dying, with the power to show loved ones and the dying a glimpse of Paradise.

Deva: nature spirit.

Emmenagogue: substance that stimulates or increases menstrual flow.

Enfleurage: extraction of essential oils and perfumes from flowers using odourless animal or vegetable fats.

Gatekeeper: these special guides act as our guardians, filtering the many energies and entities that roam the ether, challenging them if they try to enter our spiritual space.

Gatekeeper oil: this will guide and protect someone whenever they are using their consciousness outside the physical realm.

Heliotropic: directional growth of a plant or animal in response to sunlight.

Light body: the sum of a person's energetic layers, from the densest physical body to the subtlest spiritual body.

Monoterpene: present in almost all essential oils, these inhibit the accumulation of toxins and enhance the therapeutic values of other components. In effect, they balance the oils.

Myrrhophore: an ancient and secret group of women who work with the oils for the highest good of everyone.

Nous: the wisdom of the heart.

Numinous: having a strong religious or spiritual quality; indicating or suggesting the presence of a divinity.

Oleoresin: natural or artificial mixture of essential oils and a resin, such as balsam.

Oneiromancy: interpretation of dreams in order to foretell the future.

Pineal gland: a tiny mass of nerve tissue buried deep within the back of the brain and thought to be the seat of the soul and the divine connector to enlightenment within the body.

Pontiff: bridge-building priest.

Phototoxic: chemically induced skin irritation that becomes toxic after a reaction with light.

Prominence: in reference to the Sun, a stream of incandescent gas projecting above the Sun's chromosphere.

Psychopomp: an experienced practitioner who accompanies the dead for part of the way on their last journey, in order to show them the way into the beyond. This may involve being physically present when somebody dies, helping them to cross over right there and then, or at a distance.

Sigil: a sacred symbol representing energy.

Soul loss: this process happens when journeying into other dimensions, when someone unconsciously leaves a part of themselves behind in another place after failing to ground themselves properly on their return.

Soul midwife: a spiritual and holistic therapist for the dying.

Shaman: a person regarded as having access to, and influence in, the world of good and evil spirits; they practise divination and healing.

Spicule: short-lived, relatively small radial jet of gas relating to the Sun.

Thurible: a metal censer; the incense 'basket' suspended on chains and that swings through the course of a Mass. It's used as part of sacrifice and offerings, and the rising incense symbolizes prayers rising to Heaven.

Tisane: herbal, medicinal drink or infusion.

Umbelliferous: designating any plant bearing umbels – a flower cluster in which stalks of nearly equal length spring from a common centre and form a flat or curved surface.

Resources

Suggested Reading

Colour Scents: Healing with Colour and Aroma, Suzy Chiazzari (London, UK: C W Daniel Company, 1998)

Subtle Aromatherapy, Patricia Davis (Saffron Waldon, Essex, UK: C W Daniel Company, 1991)

Magical Aromatherapy: The Power of Scent, Scott Cunningham (St Paul, Minnesota: Llewellyn Publications, 1990)

The Complete Book of Incense, Oils and Brews, Scott Cunningham (St Paul, Minnesota: Llewellyn Publications, 1989)

Vibrational Medicine, Richard Gerber (Santa Fe, New Mexico: M D Bear and Co, 1998)

Mixing Essential Oils for Magic: Aromatic Alchemy for Personal Blends, Sandra Kynes (St Paul, Minnesota: Llewellyn Publications, 2013).

Sacred Luxuries: Fragrance, Aromatherapy and Cosmetics in Ancient Egypt, Lise Manniche, (London: Cornell University Press, 1999)

Aromatherapy for Healing the Spirit, Gabriel Mojay (Rochester, Vermont: Healing Arts Press, 1997)

Llewellyn's Complete Formulary of Magical Oils – Over 1200 Recipes, Potions & Tinctures for Everyday Use, Celeste Rayne Heldstab (St Paul, Minnesota: Llewellyn Publications, 2012)

The Directory of Essential Oils, Wanda Sellar (Saffron Walden, Essex: C W Daniel Company, 1992)

A Safe Journey Home, Felicity Warner (London: Hay House Publishers, 2008)

The Soul Midwives' Handbook, Felicity Warner (London: Hay House Publishers, 2013)

The Fragrant Heavens, Valerie Ann Worwood (London: Bantam Books, 1999)

Courses and Workshops

Felicity Warner runs an online course on sacred oils. Please email sacredoils@outlook.com for details of how to register.

Felicity Warner also runs workshops and retreats on sacred oils at her school in Dorset, UK and also at some other venues in the UK. Please check her website (www.soulmidwives.co.uk) for dates and other information.

Suppliers

Materia Aromatica
Essential oils, carrier oils and accessories, including glass bottles and pipettes
https://materiaaromatica.com

Oshadhi
Organic essential oils and carrier oils
https://oshadhi.co.uk

Soul Midwives
Selection of sacred oils
www.soulmidwivesshop.co.uk

Essential Oils Online
Glass bottles and pipettes
https://essentialoilsonline.co.uk

Homeopathic Supply Company
Glass bottles and labels
www.hsconline.co.uk

Bespoke Sacred Oils
Felicity Warner also creates bespoke blends for individual clients on application. Please email sacredoils@outlook.com for more information.

US Suppliers

Mountain Rose Herbs
Organic essential oils and glass bottles
https://mountainroseherbs.com

Pompeii Organics
Organic and wildcrafted essential oils and carrier oils, and glass bottles
https://pompeiiorganics.com

Young Living
Wide range of essential oils
https://youngliving.com

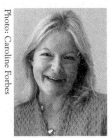

Photo: Caroline Forbes

About the Author

Felicity Warner comes from a long tradition of original thinkers dedicated to keeping perennial wisdom alive in contemporary thinking. For over 30 years, her study of philosophy, spirituality and complementary medicine has been inspired by Plato, Asclepius, Jung and the mystery traditions of both East and West.

Felicity runs the Soul Midwives School in Dorset, UK, and lectures in hospitals, hospices, universities and in the community. She combines her work and research into aromatic plant oils and their effects on the human energy field with her healing and soul ministry.

In 2017, she won the End of Life Care Champion award and the End of Life Doula award, and was a finalist in *Daily Mail* Inspirational Women of the Year awards.

www.soulmidwives.co.uk

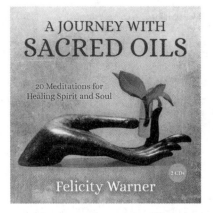

A JOURNEY WITH
SACRED OILS

20 Meditations for
Healing Spirit and Soul

2 CDs

Felicity Warner

On this meditation CD (also available as an audio download), Felicity Warner, renowned myrrhophore and soul midwife, guides you through a deep healing journey to connect with the essence of 20 sacred oils including Elemi, Holy Basil and Palo Santo.

These meditations are designed to help you connect with the ancient myrrhophore temple teachings through the lineage of Mary Magdalene. Each oil has specific properties, and has been used for thousands of years to connect with the Divine.

Through the meditations, you will:

- attune to the frequency of each oil
- heal your soul wounds and strengthen your spirit
- access sacred knowledge and past-life information
- gain knowledge of temple traditions

For anyone seeking to deepen their sacred work, this CD (or audio download) is a vital tool. The secret of the oils is known to only a handful of masters on Earth – and now, to you as well.

HAY
HOUSE

We hope you enjoyed this Hay House book. If you'd like to receive our online catalog featuring additional information on Hay House books and products, or if you'd like to find out more about the Hay Foundation, please contact:

Hay House, Inc., P.O. Box 5100, Carlsbad, CA 92018-5100
(760) 431-7695 or (800) 654-5126
(760) 431-6948 (fax) or (800) 650-5115 (fax)
www.hayhouse.com® • www.hayfoundation.org

———

Published in Australia by: Hay House Australia Pty. Ltd.,
18/36 Ralph St., Alexandria NSW 2015
Phone: 612-9669-4299 • *Fax:* 612-9669-4144
www.hayhouse.com.au

Published in the United Kingdom by: Hay House UK, Ltd.,
The Sixth Floor, Watson House, 54 Baker Street, London W1U 7BU
Phone: +44 (0)20 3927 7290 • *Fax:* +44 (0)20 3927 7291
www.hayhouse.co.uk

Published in India by: Hay House Publishers India,
Muskaan Complex, Plot No. 3, B-2, Vasant Kunj, New Delhi 110 070
Phone: 91-11-4176-1620 • *Fax:* 91-11-4176-1630
www.hayhouse.co.in

———

Access New Knowledge.
Anytime. Anywhere.

Learn and evolve at your own pace
with the world's leading experts.

www.hayhouseU.com

MEDITATE.
VISUALIZE.
LEARN.

Get the **Empower You**
Unlimited Audio *Mobile App*

Get unlimited access to the entire Hay House audio library!

You'll get:

- 500+ inspiring and life-changing **audiobooks**

- 200+ ad-free **guided meditations** for sleep, healing, relaxation, spiritual connection, and more

- Hundreds of audios **under 20 minutes** to easily fit into your day

- **Exclusive content** *only* for subscribers

- No credits, **no limits**

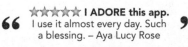
New audios added every week!

★★★★★ **I ADORE this app.** I use it almost every day. Such a blessing. – Aya Lucy Rose

Scan me with your phone camera!

TRY FOR FREE!
Go to: hayhouse.com/listen-free

HAY HOUSE
Online Video Courses

Your journey to a better life starts with figuring out which path is best for you. Hay House Online Courses provide guidance in mental and physical health, personal finance, telling your unique story, and so much more!

LEARN HOW TO:

- choose your words and actions wisely so you can tap into life's magic

- clear the energy in yourself and your environments for improved clarity, peace, and joy

- forgive, visualize, and trust in order to create a life of authenticity and abundance

- manifest lifelong health by improving nutrition, reducing stress, improving sleep, and more

- create your own unique angelic communication toolkit to help you to receive clear messages for yourself and others

- use the creative power of the quantum realm to create health and well-being

To find the guide for your journey, visit www.HayHouseU.com.

HAY HOUSE
online learning

CONNECT WITH
HAY HOUSE
ONLINE

🌐 hayhouse.co.uk   **f** @hayhouse

📷 @hayhouseuk   🐦 @hayhouseuk

▶ @hayhouseuk   ♪ @hayhouseuk

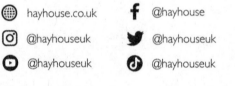

Find out all about our latest books & card decks • Be the first to know about exclusive discounts • Interact with our authors in live broadcasts • Celebrate the cycle of the seasons with us • Watch free videos from your favourite authors • Connect with like-minded souls

'The gateways to wisdom and knowledge are always open.'

Louise Hay